Emergency Airway Management

Second Edition

Emergency Airway Management

Second Edition

Edited by:

Andrew Burtenshaw
Consultant in Anaesthesia and Intensive Care Medicine, Worcestershire Acute Hospitals NHS Trust, Worcestershire, UK

Jonathan Benger
Professor of Emergency Care, University of the West of England, and Consultant in Emergency Medicine, University Hospitals Bristol NHS Foundation Trust, Bristol, UK

Jerry Nolan
Consultant in Anaesthesia and Intensive Care Medicine, Royal United Hospital, Bath, UK

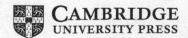

CAMBRIDGE
UNIVERSITY PRESS

CAMBRIDGE
UNIVERSITY PRESS

University Printing House, Cambridge CB2 8BS, United Kingdom

One Liberty Plaza, 20th Floor, New York, NY 10006, USA

477 Williamstown Road, Port Melbourne, VIC 3207, Australia

314-321, 3rd Floor, Plot 3, Splendor Forum, Jasola District Centre, New Delhi - 110025, India

79 Anson Road, #06-04/06, Singapore 079906

Cambridge University Press is part of the University of Cambridge.

It furthers the University's mission by disseminating knowledge in the pursuit of education, learning and research at the highest international levels of excellence.

www.cambridge.org
Information on this title: www.cambridge.org/9781107661257

© College of Emergency Medicine, London, 2015

First published 2008
Second edition 2015
3rd printing 2016

A catalogue record for this publication is available from the British Library

ISBN 978-1-107-66125-7 Paperback

Cambridge University Press has no responsibility for the persistence or accuracy of URLs for external or third-party internet websites referred to in this publication, and does not guarantee that any content on such websites is, or will remain, accurate or appropriate.

....

Every effort has been made in preparing this book to provide accurate and up-to-date information which is in accord with accepted standards and practice at the time of publication. Although case histories are drawn from actual cases, every effort has been made to disguise the identities of the individuals involved. Nevertheless, the authors, editors and publishers can make no warranties that the information contained herein is totally free from error, not least because clinical standards are constantly changing through research and regulation. The authors, editors and publishers therefore disclaim all liability for direct or consequential damages resulting from the use of material contained in this book. Readers are strongly advised to pay careful attention to information provided by the manufacturer of any drugs or equipment that they plan to use.

Contents

Contributors

Jonathan Benger MD FRCS FCEM
Professor of Emergency Care,
University of the West of England,
and Consultant in Emergency
Medicine, University Hospitals Bristol
NHS Foundation Trust, Bristol, UK

**John C. Berridge MB ChB
FRCPEdin FRCA FFICM**
Consultant in Anaesthesia and
Intensive Care Medicine, York
Teaching Hospitals NHS
Foundation Trust, York, UK

**Andrew Burtenshaw MBChB
MRCP FRCA FFICM**
Consultant in Anaesthesia and
Intensive Care Medicine,
Worcestershire Acute
Hospitals NHS Trust,
Worcestershire, UK

Stephen Bush MD
Consultant in Emergency Medicine,
Leeds Teaching Hospitals Trust,
Leeds, UK

**Simon J. A. Chapman MBBS
BMedSci FRCS(AE) Ed FCEM**
Consultant in Emergency Medicine,
Jersey General Hospital, St Helier,
Jersey, UK

John Clift MBChB FRCA
Consultant in Anaesthesia and
Critical Care Medicine, Sandwell
and West Birmingham Hospitals
NHS Trust, Birmingham, UK

Tim Cook BA MBBS FRCA FFICM
Professor and Consultant in
Anaesthesia and Intensive Care
Medicine, Royal United Hospital,
Bath, UK

Kevin J. Fong MSc MRCP FRCA
Consultant Anaesthetist, University
College London Hospitals,
London, UK

Chris Frerk FRCA
Consultant Anaesthetist,
Northampton General Hospital,
Northampton, UK

**Dinendra S. Gill BmedSci MBChB
MRCS (RCS Eng) Dip IMC (RCS
Ed) FCEM**
Consultant in Emergency
Medicine, Morriston Hospital,
Swansea, UK

Les Gordon MB ChB FRCA
Consultant Anaesthetist,
Morecambe Bay University
Hospitals Trust, Lancaster, and
Team Doctor, Langdale Ambleside
Mountain Rescue Team,
Cumbria, UK

**Colin A. Graham MB ChB MPH
MD FRCPEd FRCSEd FRCSGlasg
FIMCRCSEd FCCP FCEM
FHKCEM FHKAM (Emergency
Medicine)**
Professor of Emergency Medicine
and Honorary Consultant in

Emergency Medicine, Chinese University of Hong Kong and Prince of Wales Hospital, Shatin, New Territories, Hong Kong

Carl Gwinnutt MB BS FRCA
Emeritus Consultant in Anaesthesia, Salford Royal Hospital Foundation Trust, Salford, UK

Jonathan Hulme MBChB MRCP FRCA DipIMC FFICM
Consultant in Intensive Care Medicine and Anaesthesia, Sandwell and West Birmingham Hospitals NHS Trust; Honorary Senior Clinical Lecturer, Unversity of Birmingham, Birmingham; West Midlands Ambulance Service NHS Foundation Trust Medical Emergency Response Incident Team (MERIT); Director, West Midlands Central Accident Resuscitation Emergency (CARE) Team; Mercia Accident Rescue Service (MARS) BASICS, UK

Shirley Lindsay MBChB FRCA
Consultant Anaesthetist, Worcestershire Royal Hospital, Worcestershire Acute Hospitals NHS Trust, Worcester, UK

Gavin Lloyd MBBS FRCS(EM) FCEM
Consultant in Emergency Medicine, Royal Devon & Exeter Hospital, Devon, UK

Dermot McKeown FRCA FFICM
Consultant in Anaesthesia and Critical Care, Royal Infirmary of Edinburgh, Edinburgh, UK

Jerry Nolan FRCA FRCP FFICM FCEM (Hon)
Consultant in Anaesthesia and Intensive Care Medicine, Royal United Hospital, Bath, UK

Gavin Perkins MB ChB MD MMEd FRCP FFICM FERC
Professor of Critical Care Medicine, University of Warwick, Coventry, and Consultant in Intensive Care, Heart of England NHS Foundation Trust, Birmingham, UK

David Ray MD MBChB FRCA FFICM
Consultant in Anaesthesia and Critical Care, Royal Infirmary of Edinburgh, Edinburgh, UK

Patricia Weir FRCA FRCPCH
Consultant in Paediatric Anaesthesia and Intensive Care, Bristol Royal Hospital for Children, Bristol, UK

Dominic Williamson BM MRCP DA FCEM
Consultant in Emergency Medicine, Royal University Hospital Bath, Bath, UK

Nick Woodall MB ChB FRCA
Consultant Anaesthetist, Norfolk and Norwich University Hospitals NHS Foundation Trust, Norfolk, UK

Paul Younge DA MRCP FCEM FACEM
Consultant in Emergency Medicine, Frenchay Hospital, North Bristol NHS Trust, Bristol, UK

Foreword

When the first edition of this book was published in 2008 it heralded a new approach to the way in which management of the airway in emergency situations was taught. The emphasis was placed firmly on competency rather than specialty. Both the book and the course it accompanies have achieved considerable success, delivering a didactic yet pragmatic approach to the management of the compromised airway.

As ever competence can only be achieved through both the acquisition of knowledge and practical skills and can only be maintained through regular practice and experiential learning. This book is a companion to these endeavours but not a substitute.

The essence of safe airway management is the decision-making process that achieves safety with effectiveness, thereby minimizing iatrogenic error whilst attaining airway security and optimizing ventilation and oxygenation.

The book lays the foundations for achieving these competencies with clear and concise descriptions of the anatomy, physiology and pharmacology of emergency airway management. This is complemented by discussions on the detailed management of some commonly encountered clinical scenarios.

The book has been extensively updated and revised since the first edition and now contains a new chapter examining the importance and influence of non-technical human factors. The introduction of and more widespread use of videolaryngoscopy is reflected by a description and discussion of its role as an aid to airway management. Also of major significance is the fact that the book now reflects the findings and conclusions of the National Audit of Major Airway Complications in the UK published in 2011 (NAP4).

The book should be an essential accompaniment to any trainee involved in the acute care of the patient with a potentially compromised airway including anaesthetists, emergency physicians and acute physicians in a variety of environments from pre-hospital care through to the emergency department, operating room and critical care unit.

Dr Clifford Mann FRCP FCEM
President, College of Emergency Medicine

Dr J-P van Besouw BSc (Hons) MBBS FRCA FRCP Ed Hon FRCS
President, Royal College of Anaesthetists

Note

This book and the course it accompanies have been prepared by a group of clinicians from the specialties of anaesthesia, intensive care and emergency medicine.

The UK TEAM Course, this manual and all course materials are the intellectual property of these individuals, who are listed in the contributor list. However, the course has been developed and refined by the group as a whole, through a process of ongoing discussion and collaboration.

The rights of the Authors to be identified as the Authors of this Work have been asserted in accordance with the Copyright, Designs and Patents Act 1988.

This manual has been edited by Andrew Burtenshaw, Jonathan Benger and Jerry Nolan, to whom all comments should be addressed.

July 2014

Department of Anaesthesia and Intensive Care Medicine
Worcestershire Royal Hospital
Worcester, WR5 1DD
Andrew.Burtenshaw@worcsacute.nhs.uk

Academic Department of Emergency Care,
Bristol Royal Infirmary, Bristol, BS2 8HW
Jonathan.Benger@UHBristol.nhs.uk

Department of Anaesthesia and Intensive Care Medicine
Royal United Hospital
Bath, BA1 3NG
Jerry.nolan@nhs.net

Abbreviations

ABCD Airway, breathing, circulation and disability
ANTS Anaesthetic non-technical skills
APL Adjustable pressure limiting (valve)
ARDS Acute respiratory distress syndrome
ATLS Advanced trauma life support
BMI Body mass index
BMV Bag-mask ventilation
BTS British Thoracic Society
BURP Backwards, upwards, rightwards pressure
CICO Can't intubate, can't oxygenate
CMV Continuous mandatory ventilation
CO_2 Carbon dioxide
COPD Chronic obstructive pulmonary disease
CPAP Continuous positive airway pressure
CPP Cerebral perfusion pressure
CPR Cardiopulmonary resuscitation
CSI Cervical spine injury
CT Computed tomography
ECG Electrocardiograph
ED Emergency department
ENT Ear, nose and throat
EPAP Expiratory positive airway pressure
E_TCO_2 End tidal carbon dioxide
FEV_1 Forced expiratory volume over one second
FG French gauge
FGF Fresh gas flow
F_iO_2 Inspired oxygen concentration
FRC Functional residual capacity
GABA Gamma-amino butyric acid
GCS Glasgow Coma Scale

HAFOE High-airflow oxygen enrichment
HME Heat and moisture exchanger
ICNARC Intensive Care National Audit And Research Centre
ICP Intracranial pressure
ICU Intensive care unit
ILMA Intubating laryngeal mask airway
IOP Intraocular pressure
IPAP Inspiratory positive airway pressure
IPPV Intermittent positive pressure ventilation
LED Light-emitting diode
LMA Laryngeal mask airway
MAP Mean arterial pressure
MET Medical emergency team
MMC Modernizing medical careers
MV Minute volume
NAP4 Fourth National Audit Project of the Royal College of Anaesthetists and the Intensive Care Society
NEAR National Emergency Airway Registry
NIBP Non-invasive blood pressure
NICE National Institute for Health and Care Excellence
NIPPV Non-invasive positive pressure ventilation
NIV Non-invasive ventilation
NMJ Neuromuscular junction
NTSP National Tracheostomy Safety Project
O_2 Oxygen
P_ACO_2 Partial pressure of carbon dioxide (alveolar)
P_AO_2 Partial pressure of oxygen (alveolar)

P_aCO_2 Partial pressure of carbon dioxide (arterial)

P_aO_2 Partial pressure of oxygen (arterial)

PEEP Positive end expiratory pressure

PICU Paediatric intensive care unit

PLMA ProSeal laryngeal mask airway

P_{max} Peak (maximum) inspiratory pressure

PO_2 Partial pressure of oxygen

$\dot{Q}$ Perfusion

RR Respiratory rate

RSI Rapid sequence induction (of anaesthesia)

SAD Supraglottic airway device

SBAR Situation, Background, Assessment, Recommendation

SIGN Scottish Intercollegiate Guidelines Network

SIMV Synchronized intermittent mandatory ventilation

S_aO_2 Oxygen saturation (arterial)

S_pO_2 Oxygen saturation by pulse oximetry

TBI Traumatic brain injury

TRM Team resource management

$\dot{V}$ Ventilation

$\dot{V}/\dot{Q}$ Ventilation/Perfusion ratio

VALI Ventilator associated lung injury

V_T Tidal volume

Chapter 1

Introduction

Andrew Burtenshaw, Jonathan Benger and Jerry Nolan

Introduction

Effective airway management is central to the care of critically ill and injured patients. Competency in assessment and maintenance of the airway using basic airway manoeuvres first, followed by advanced skills such as rapid sequence induction of anaesthesia and tracheal intubation, are core skills for doctors who treat seriously ill or potentially ill patients. In the UK, this typically involves the specialties of:

- anaesthesia;
- emergency medicine;
- intensive care medicine.

The location for emergency airway management is usually outside the relatively controlled environment of an anaesthetic room, most commonly in the resuscitation room of an emergency department, but also in a variety of other in-hospital and pre-hospital settings. Emergency airway management can be difficult and challenging; it requires individuals to work in relatively unfamiliar environments under conditions of stress and uncertainty, and where the principles of elective anaesthesia need modification. Information is often incomplete, normal physiology deranged, and opportunity for delay is infrequent. The problems intrinsic to these patients, such as an unstable cervical spine, poor cardiorespiratory reserve or profound metabolic dysfunction, must be anticipated and surmounted.

Emergency airway management is not simply an extension of elective anaesthesia, and specific training is essential to safely treat this challenging and heterogeneous group of patients. Individuals must practice within the limits of their own competence and work collaboratively with experienced clinicians from several disciplines to ensure patients receive optimal care (Figure 1.1).

Emergency Airway Management, Second Edition, ed. Andrew Burtenshaw, Jonathan Benger and Jerry Nolan. Published by Cambridge University Press. © College of Emergency Medicine, London, 2015.

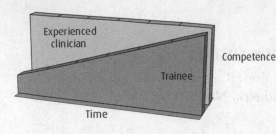

Figure 1.1
A collaborative
approach ensures
the best patient care.

Competence

Experienced
clinician

Trainee

Time

Skills and judgement, as well as knowledge, are essential for treating patients who require emergency airway intervention. Careful judgement is required to determine whether an intervention is appropriate, how and when it should be undertaken, and what additional personnel and equipment are needed.

Central to emergency airway management is the recognition of:

1. The fundamental importance of good basic airways skills.
2. The need for close collaboration with those who are already competent to enable effective clinical training. It is essential to work alongside practitioners who have established expertise in emergency airway care in order to build upon and apply theoretical learning. A clinician working alone should not attempt emergency airway interventions that are outside the limits of their own competence.

The second edition of this book addresses the rapidly changing landscape of emergency airway management outside the operating room. Widespread access to technologies such as videolaryngoscopy, updated guidance based on emerging clinical evidence and increasing recognition of the role of human factors are just some of the elements that have shaped changes in clinical practice, and the second edition reflects these.

Audit and skills maintenance

Audit and peer review of clinical practice must be undertaken continuously to ensure standards are maintained. Medical simulators are becoming more sophisticated, and have a valuable role in the development, retention and assessment of clinical skills and human factors.

Summary

- This manual will not provide competence in emergency airway management, but offers a firm foundation upon which further training and assessment can be based.
- Effective emergency airway management requires commitment to a process of ongoing training, assessment, skill maintenance and audit that will last throughout the practitioner's professional career.

Delivery of oxygen

Carl Gwinnutt

2

Objectives

The objectives of this chapter are to:

- Understand the causes of hypoxaemia.
- Understand how much oxygen to give.
- Be familiar with devices that enable an increase in the inspired oxygen concentration.
- Understand the function and use of the self-inflating bag-mask.
- Understand the function and use of the Mapleson C breathing system.
- Understand how to monitor oxygenation.
- Understand the principle of pre-oxygenation.

Causes of hypoxaemia

The strict definition of hypoxaemia is a partial pressure of oxygen in the arterial blood (P_aO_2) below normal. For patients with no respiratory pathology, a value of <8 kPa or 60 mmHg (equivalent to an arterial oxygen saturation of approximately 90%) is often used to define hypoxaemia requiring treatment; for patients with chronic obstructive pulmonary disease (COPD), a P_aO_2 <8 kPa (S_pO_2 <90%) may be 'normal'. In nearly all patients hypoxaemia can usually be improved, at least initially, by increasing the inspired oxygen concentration.

Although the cause of hypoxaemia is usually multifactorial, there are several distinct mechanisms:

- alveolar hypoventilation;
- mismatch between ventilation and perfusion within the lungs;
- pulmonary diffusion abnormalities;
- reduced inspired oxygen concentration.

Emergency Airway Management, Second Edition, ed. Andrew Burtenshaw, Jonathan Benger and Jerry Nolan. Published by Cambridge University Press. © College of Emergency Medicine, London, 2015.

Alveolar hypoventilation

If insufficient oxygen enters the alveoli to replace that taken up by the blood, both the alveolar (P_AO_2) and arterial (P_aO_2) partial pressure of oxygen decrease. In most patients, increasing the inspired oxygen concentration will restore both. When an adult's tidal volume decreases below approximately 150 mL there is no ventilation of the alveoli, only the 'dead space', which is the volume of the airways that plays no part in gas exchange. No oxygen reaches the alveoli, irrespective of the inspired concentration, and profound hypoxaemia will follow. At this point ventilatory support **and** supplementary oxygen will be required. Hypoventilation is always accompanied by hypercapnia, as there is an inverse relationship between arterial partial pressure of carbon dioxide (P_aCO_2) and alveolar ventilation.

Common causes of hypoventilation are as follows:

Airway obstruction:

- tongue;
- blood;
- vomit;
- bronchospasm;
- oedema (infection, burns, allergy).

Central respiratory depression:

- drugs;
- alcohol;
- central nervous system injury (cerebrovascular event, trauma, etc.);
- hypothermia.

Impaired mechanics of ventilation:

- pain;
- pneumothorax or flail chest;
- haemothorax;
- pulmonary oedema;
- diaphragmatic splinting;
- pre-existing lung disease.

Mismatch between ventilation and perfusion within the lungs

Normally, ventilation of the alveoli ($\dot{V}$) and perfusion with blood ($\dot{Q}$) are well matched ($\dot{V}/\dot{Q} = 1$), ensuring that haemoglobin in blood leaving the lungs is saturated with oxygen (Figure 2.1). If this process is disturbed ($\dot{V}/\dot{Q}$ mismatch) regions develop where:

1. Ventilation is less than perfusion ($\dot{V}/\dot{Q}<1$), resulting in haemoglobin with reduced oxygen content, e.g. pneumothorax, pneumonia.

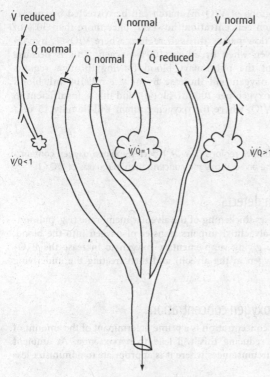

Figure 2.1 Different $\dot{V}/\dot{Q}$ ratios.

Reduced oxygen content

2. Perfusion is less than ventilation ($\dot{V}/\dot{Q} > 1$). This can be considered wasted ventilation as very little additional oxygen is taken up when haemoglobin is already almost fully saturated (98%), e.g. hypotension, pulmonary embolus.

At its most extreme, some regions of the lung may be perfused but not ventilated ($\dot{V}/\dot{Q} = 0$); blood leaving these areas remains 'venous', and is often referred to as shunted blood. This is then mixed with oxygenated blood leaving ventilated regions of the lungs. The final oxygen content of blood leaving the lungs is dependent on the relative proportions of blood from these two regions:

- Blood perfusing ventilated alveoli leaves with an oxygen content of approximately 20 mL/100 mL blood (assuming a haemoglobin concentration of 150 gL^{-1}).
- Blood perfusing unventilated alveoli remains 'venous', leaving with an oxygen content of 15 mL/100 mL blood.

The effect of small regions of $\dot{V}/\dot{Q}$ mismatch can be corrected by increasing the inspired oxygen concentration; however, once more than 30% of the pulmonary blood flow passes through regions where $\dot{V}/\dot{Q}<1$, hypoxaemia is inevitable, even when breathing 100% oxygen. This is because the oxygen content of the pulmonary blood flowing through regions ventilated with 100% oxygen will increase by only 1 mL/100 mL blood (to produce 21 mL of oxygen per 100 mL blood), and this is insufficient to offset regions of low $\dot{V}/\dot{Q}$, where the oxygen content will be only 15 mL/100 mL blood.

> For an equivalent blood flow, regions of $\dot{V}/\dot{Q}<1$ decrease blood oxygen content more than increasing the alveolar oxygen concentration in regions of $\dot{V}/\dot{Q}>1$.

Pulmonary diffusion defects

Any condition that causes thickening of the alveolar membrane (e.g. pulmonary oedema, fibrosing alveolitis) impairs transfer of oxygen into the blood. This is treated first by giving supplementary oxygen to increase the P_AO_2 (partial pressure of oxygen in the alveoli) and then treating the underlying problem.

A reduced inspired oxygen concentration

As the inspired oxygen concentration is a prime determinant of the amount of oxygen in the alveoli, reducing this will lead to hypoxaemia. At ambient pressure there are no circumstances where it is appropriate to administer less than 21% oxygen.

How much oxygen?

In the past, oxygen has usually been given on the basis that if some is good, more must be better. It is now recognized that in most circumstances, there is a range of optimal oxygenation and in some conditions (e.g. post-acute myocardial infarction, ischaemic stroke), excess oxygen may be detrimental. In 2008, the British Thoracic Society (BTS) published 'Guidelines for Emergency Oxygen Use in Adult Patients'. These guidelines recommend that for most acutely ill patients, oxygen should be given to achieve a target saturation of 94–98%, or 88–92% for those at risk of hypercapnic respiratory failure.

Give all critically ill patients (Table 2.1) high-flow oxygen (15 L min⁻¹) until they are stable; then reduce the inspired oxygen concentration to achieve a target saturation of 94–98%. Patients with COPD and other risk factors for hypercapnic respiratory failure who are critically ill are treated similarly, but

Table 2.1 Critically ill patients

- Cardiac arrest or peri-arrest resuscitation
- Shock
- Sepsis
- Near-drowning
- Anaphylaxis
- Major pulmonary haemorrhage
- Major head injury
- Carbon monoxide poisoning

aim for a saturation of 88–92% once they are stable. When pulse oximetry is unavailable, give high-flow oxygen until definitive treatment is available.

Early assessment of gas exchange based on the analysis of an arterial blood sample is essential in all critically ill patients to guide the need for subsequent oxygen therapy or ventilatory support.

Whenever oxygen is given to a patient, it must be prescribed and the target oxygen saturation to be maintained written on the patient's drug chart.

Devices used for delivery of oxygen

Spontaneous ventilation

Variable-performance devices: masks or nasal cannulae

With these devices, the precise concentration of oxygen inspired by the patient is unknown, because it depends on the patient's respiratory pattern and the oxygen flow (usually 2–15 L min^{-1}). When breathing through a mask the inspired gas consists of a mixture of:

- oxygen flowing into the mask;
- oxygen that has accumulated under the mask during the expiratory pause;
- alveolar gas exhaled during the previous breath that has collected under the mask;
- air entrained during inspiration from the holes in the side of the mask and from leaks between the mask and face.

An example of this type of device is the Hudson mask (Figure 2.2). As a guide, the inspired oxygen concentration will be 25–60% with oxygen flows of 2–15 L min^{-1}. Patients unable to tolerate a facemask, but who can nose breathe, may find either a single foam-tipped catheter or double catheters, placed just inside the vestibule of the nose, more comfortable (Figure 2.3). Lower flows of oxygen are used; 2–4 L min^{-1} increases the inspired oxygen concentration to 25–40%.

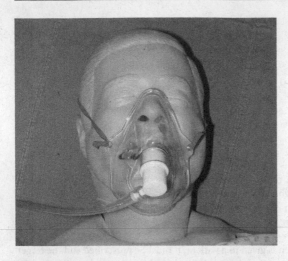

Figure 2.2
Hudson mask.

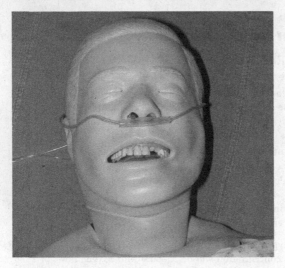

Figure 2.3 Nasal cannulae.

In a critically ill patient breathing spontaneously who requires a higher concentration of oxygen, a Hudson mask with a reservoir (non-rebreathing bag) can be used (Figure 2.4). A one-way valve diverts the oxygen flow into the reservoir during expiration. During inspiration, the contents of the reservoir,

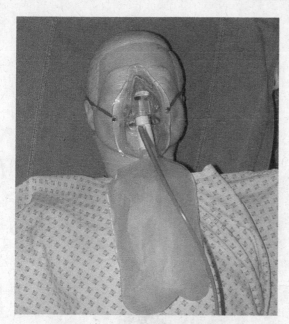

Figure 2.4 Hudson mask with reservoir.

along with the high flow of oxygen (12–15 L min^{-1}), ensure minimal entrainment of air, raising the inspired concentration to approximately 80%, providing that the reservoir bag inflates and deflates with each breath. This requires a well-fitting, functioning mask and reservoir, and is often overlooked in clinical practice. An inspired oxygen concentration of 100% can be achieved only by using a close-fitting facemask with an anaesthetic breathing system that includes a reservoir, combined with an oxygen flow of 12–15 L min^{-1} (see below). Once stable, these patients should have oxygen therapy adjusted as described above.

Fixed-performance devices

These are used to deliver a precise concentration of oxygen, unaffected by the patient's ventilatory pattern. These devices work on the principle of high-airflow oxygen enrichment (HAFOE). Oxygen is delivered to a Venturi that entrains a much greater, but constant, flow of air (Figure 2.5). The total flow into the mask needs to be as high as 45 L min^{-1}. The high gas flow has two effects: it exceeds the patient's peak inspiratory flow, reducing entrainment of air, and flushes expiratory gas, reducing rebreathing. These are the devices of choice for patients with known hypercapnic respiratory failure, or who are at risk of this condition.

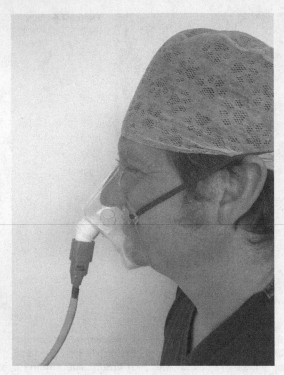

Figure 2.5 Use of a HAFOE mask delivering (in this case) 40% oxygen.

These devices deliver a fixed concentration for a given flow, and there are several interchangeable Venturis to vary the oxygen concentration (Table 2.2).

The above systems all deliver dry gas to the patient, which may cause crusting or thickening of secretions, difficulty with clearance, and patient discomfort. For prolonged use, a HAFOE system should be used with a humidifier.

Assisted ventilation

Patients whose ventilation is inadequate to maintain oxygenation despite an increase in the inspired oxygen concentration using one of the devices described above, or who are apnoeic, will require oxygenation using a mechanical device. The simplest and most widely used device is the bag-mask (Figure 2.6). An alternative is an anaesthetic breathing system (Figure 2.9).

Table 2.2 Effect of type of Venturi valve and oxygen flow on inspired oxygen concentration.

Venturi valve colour	Oxygen flow (L min^{-1})	Inspired oxygen concentration (%)
Blue	2	24
White	4	28
Yellow	6	35
Red	8	40
Green	12	60

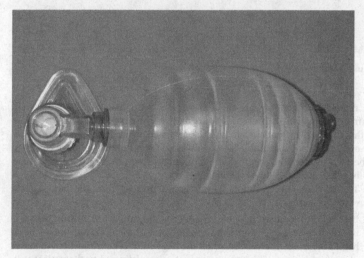

Figure 2.6 Self-inflating bag-mask.

In selected patients improved oxygenation, as well as ventilatory assistance, can be achieved using either continuous positive airway pressure (CPAP) or non-invasive positive pressure ventilation (NiPPV). These forms of non-invasive ventilatory support are described in Chapter 12.

The bag-mask device

In its simplest form this consists of a self-inflating bag; when squeezed, the contents are delivered to the patient via a non-return valve and facemask.

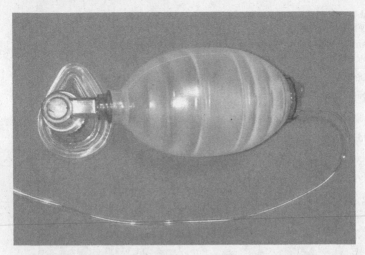

Figure 2.7 Bag-mask with oxygen attached.

On release, the bag entrains air as it returns to its original shape. Expired air from the patient is prevented from reaching the bag by a one-way valve. In this manner, the patient's lungs are ventilated with air (21% oxygen). The use of clear, plastic disposable facemasks enable regurgitated stomach contents to be seen sooner and 'fogging' of the plastic during exhalation indicates that gas is going into and out of the lungs.

The oxygen concentration in the gas delivered from the bag can be increased in two ways:

1. By connecting a high flow of oxygen (10–15 L min^{-1}) to an inlet port, usually adjacent to the air entrainment valve at the opposite end of the bag to the mask. In this way, when the bag refills, it does so with a mixture of air and oxygen. The oxygen concentration delivered to the patient will depend upon several factors including oxygen flow, rate of ventilation and volume delivered. In the average adult, the concentration is unlikely to exceed 50% (Figure 2.7).

2. In addition to the above, a reservoir can be attached over the air entrainment valve. As the bag is squeezed to ventilate the patient's lungs, the oxygen flow is diverted and accumulates within the reservoir. As the bag is released it refills from the contents of the reservoir and the oxygen flow, thereby virtually eliminating air entrainment. In this manner, providing the oxygen flow exceeds the minute ventilation of the lungs, close to 100% oxygen can be delivered (Figure 2.8).

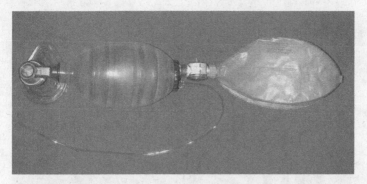

Figure 2.8 Bag-mask with oxygen and reservoir.

Oxygen delivery with this device in any configuration is dependent on:

1. The practitioner being able to maintain a good seal between the facemask and the patient's face, so that there is minimal escape of gas around the mask when the bag is squeezed. This is best achieved by using a two-person technique: one holds the facemask with both hands, while the other squeezes the bag.
2. Avoidance of high pressure and excessive volumes to ventilate the patient's lungs; these result in gas being forced down the oesophagus and into the stomach. This will reduce ventilation of the lungs and predispose to regurgitation and aspiration.

The commonest reason for requiring high pressures to ventilate the patient's lungs is failure to maintain a patent airway. This is commonly caused by:

1. Poor airway control: this can often be overcome by using a two-person technique.
2. Foreign material in the airway, e.g. vomit, blood: this must be removed using a safe and effective suction technique.

Although a patient can breathe oxygen spontaneously from a bag-mask device, this is suboptimal because effort is needed to overcome the resistance to inspiratory and expiratory flow. Spontaneously breathing patients should be given oxygen using one of the devices described above, or via an anaesthetic breathing system.

The anaesthetic breathing system

This can be used during both spontaneous and assisted ventilation. Safe use requires an understanding of function, which differs depending on whether the patient is breathing spontaneously or ventilation is assisted.

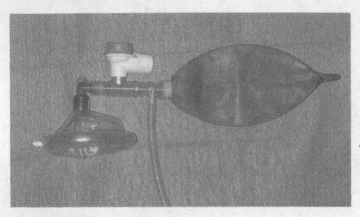

Figure 2.9 Mapleson C anaesthetic breathing system.

The most commonly used system in emergency airway management is the Mapleson C breathing system (Figure 2.9). It comprises:

1. An oxygen input, either from the common gas outlet of an anaesthetic machine or a wall-mounted flowmeter.
2. A reservoir bag. This has several functions:
   a. It collects the inflowing oxygen during expiration, which is then used to meet the patient's peak inspiratory flow during spontaneous ventilation.
   b. Movement of the bag can be used as an indicator of ventilation.
   c. It can be squeezed to deliver oxygen to assist ventilation.
   d. If the expiratory valve is closed (or blocked) excess gas accumulates in the bag with minimal increase in airway pressure (a safety feature to protect the patient's lungs from barotrauma).
3. An adjustable, pressure limiting (APL) valve usually referred to as the expiratory valve. This opens during expiration to enable the escape of exhaled gas (containing carbon dioxide) and prevent its accumulation within the system. This valve also enables the escape of any surplus oxygen flow. The valve can be adjusted manually from fully open (minimal opening pressure) to fully closed (no gas escape is possible through the valve).
4. A connection to a facemask: this is often a short, flexible piece of tubing that may incorporate a bacterial filter.

An important feature of this system is the potential for accumulation of exhaled carbon dioxide within the reservoir bag, which will result in significant hypercapnia. To prevent this, the gas flow must exceed twice the patient's minute volume. Always use a minimum oxygen flow of 12–15 L min^{-1}.

Using the Mapleson C breathing system

Spontaneous ventilation The mask is held on the patient's face with the expiratory valve fully open so that expiration is unimpeded. As the patient breathes in, the negative pressure closes the valve and the bag will collapse slightly. During expiration, the oxygen flow refills the bag and flushes out the exhaled gas containing CO_2, resulting in an audible leak of gas via the valve.

Assisted ventilation The mask is held on the patient's face and the expiratory valve manually adjusted (partially closed) so that sufficient pressure can be generated by squeezing the bag to inflate the lungs (this will often require a second person). Some gas will be heard escaping via the valve. During expiration, the oxygen flow refills the bag and flushes out the exhaled gas containing CO_2, resulting in an audible leak of gas via the valve. If the valve is not closed sufficiently during attempted ventilation, the oxygen escapes via the valve rather than entering the patient's lungs.

Pitfalls when using an anaesthetic breathing system

Spontaneous ventilation

1. Inadequate oxygen flow. Carbon dioxide is not flushed from the system and accumulates in the bag. This leads to rebreathing and the patient will become hypercapnoeic with several adverse effects, e.g. increased cerebral blood flow and intracranial pressure, cardiac arrhythmias.
2. Expiratory valve closed. This prevents expiration, causing an increase in intrathoracic pressure that may have several serious consequences, e.g. increasing intracranial pressure, barotrauma. Gas may also be forced into the stomach and predispose to abdominal splinting and regurgitation. In practice, either an increasing leak develops around the mask or the distending bag should alert the practitioner.

Assisted ventilation

1. Inadequate oxygen flow. It becomes increasingly difficult to provide adequate ventilation as the bag gradually collapses. At this point, the danger is that the expiratory valve is gradually closed to prevent escape of gas and maintain enough volume in the system to squeeze the bag. Although this will apparently enable the patient's lungs to be ventilated, carbon dioxide is not eliminated and accumulates within the system. The patient becomes rapidly hypercapnoeic, with the problems described above.

Because of the specialist nature of anaesthetic breathing systems, only those with appropriate training should use them.

Monitoring oxygenation

The pulse oximeter

A probe, containing a light-emitting diode (LED) and a photo-detector, is applied across the tip of a digit or earlobe. The LED emits red light alternately at two different wavelengths, in the visible and infrared regions of the electromagnetic spectrum. These are transmitted through the tissues and absorbed to different degrees by oxyhaemoglobin and deoxyhaemoglobin. The intensity of light reaching the photo-detector is converted to an electrical signal. The absorption by the tissues and venous blood is static. This is then subtracted from the beat-to-beat variation in absorption due to arterial blood to display the peripheral arterial oxygen saturation (S_pO_2), both as a waveform and a digital reading. Pulse oximeters are accurate to ±2% for values in excess of 70%. Below this their accuracy is poorly validated. The waveform can also indicate the heart rate. Alarms are provided for arterial blood saturation and heart rate values. The pulse oximeter therefore gives information about both the circulatory and respiratory systems, and has the advantages of:

- providing continuous monitoring of oxygenation at tissue level;
- being unaffected by skin pigmentation;
- portability (mains or battery powered);
- being non-invasive.

There are several important limitations to this device:

- Failure to realize the severity of hypoxaemia; because of the shape of the oxyhaemoglobin dissociation curve (Figure 2.10), a saturation of 90% equates to a P_aO_2 of 8 kPa (60 mmHg).
- Unreliable when there is severe vasoconstriction, because of the reduced pulsatile component of the signal.
- Provides no indication of the P_aCO_2; profound hypercapnia is possible with normal oxygen saturations, particularly in the presence of alveolar hypoventilation and a high concentration of inspired oxygen.
- Unreliable with certain haemoglobins:
  a. when carboxyhaemoglobin is present, it overestimates arterial oxygen saturation (S_aO_2)
  b. when methaemoglobin is present, at saturations greater than 85% it underestimates S_aO_2.
- Progressively under-reads the saturation as the haemoglobin decreases (but is not affected by polycythaemia).
- Affected by extraneous light.
- Unreliable when there is excessive movement of the patient.

The pulse oximeter is not an indicator of the adequacy of alveolar ventilation.

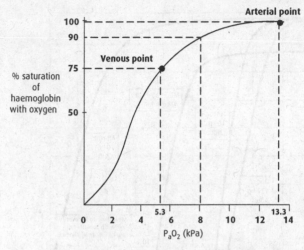

Figure 2.10 *The oxygen–haemoglobin dissociation curve.* The shape of the oxygen–haemoglobin dissociation curve indicates that the oxygen saturation of blood decreases rapidly below 92%; therefore, when the oxygen saturation displayed on the pulse oximeter decreases to 92%, corrective action is required, and the patient should be reoxygenated immediately.

Arterial blood gas analysis

The analysis of an arterial blood gas sample is essential for assessing the adequacy of oxygenation and ventilation. Information on the interpretation of arterial blood gases can be found in the further reading section.

Pre-oxygenation

Effective pre-oxygenation enables several minutes of apnoea without desaturation of arterial blood, during which tracheal intubation can be achieved. An oxygen reservoir is developed by replacing air (nitrogen) in the lungs (the functional residual capacity) with oxygen, and saturating the blood and tissues. One of the most efficient ways of achieving this is by giving 100% oxygen via a Mapleson C breathing system. A bag-mask device is a less suitable alternative because of the resistance to inspiratory and expiratory flow, and the inability to deliver 100% oxygen. An oxygen mask with a properly functioning reservoir bag delivers approximately 80% oxygen and is an alternative, although less effective, method if an anaesthetic breathing system is not immediately available, or the patient will not tolerate a well-fitting facemask. The efficiency of pre-oxygenation can be further optimized by the use of CPAP, which may be

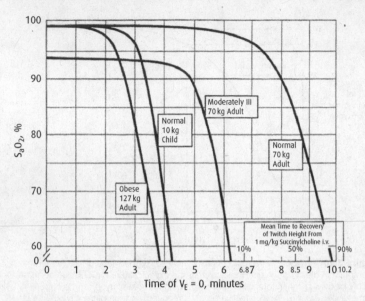

Figure 2.11 *Time to desaturation according to a range of patient characteristics.*
Time to haemoglobin desaturation with initial F_AO_2=0.87 for various patient
circumstances. Note the bars indicating recovery from succinylcholine paralysis at
the bottom right of the graph. (From Benumof, J., Dagg, R., Benumof, R. (1997)
Critical hemoglobin desaturation will occur before return to an unparalyzed state
following 1 mg kg^{-1} intravenous succinylcholine. *Anesthesiology*; **87**: 979–82,
with permission.)

delivered by adjusting the APL valve of the Mapleson C system. This may be
of particular benefit for patients with severe lung disease, where use of high-
flow continuous positive airway pressure (CPAP) for pre-oxygenation will
enable the highest possible arterial blood oxygen saturation to be achieved.

The time for arterial blood to desaturate is related to the effectiveness of
the pre-oxygenation phase, the age and weight of the patient, and the patient's
physiological status. In a healthy adult following effective pre-oxygenation, the
time for arterial blood to desaturate to 92% may be as long as eight minutes;
for a child, this is reduced to four minutes. All these times are reduced in an
ill patient, who is usually unable to achieve full pre-oxygenation, especially if
ventilation is inadequate (Figure 2.11). Once the saturation reaches 92%, the
rate of desaturation accelerates because of the shape of the oxyhaemoglobin
dissociation curve (Figure 2.10).

Summary

- The commonest causes of hypoxaemia are hypoventilation and ventilation/perfusion mismatch, both of which can be managed initially by increasing the inspired oxygen concentration.
- Target oxygen therapy according to the patient's needs and prescribe appropriately.
- A variety of devices are available to deliver oxygen in patients breathing spontaneously or requiring assisted ventilation.
- The pulse oximeter provides a useful indication of arterial oxygenation, but not the adequacy of ventilation.
- Pre-oxygenation is an important step in preparing for rapid sequence induction, and is achieved best by using an anaesthetic breathing system or, in some cases, CPAP.

Further reading

1 West, J.B. (2011) *Respiratory Physiology: The Essentials*, 9th edn. Philadelphia: Lippincott, Williams and Wilkins.

2 Nolan, J., Soar, J., Lockey, A. *et al.* (eds.). (2011) *Advanced Life Support*, 6th edn. London: Resuscitation Council.

3 Gwinnutt, C., Gwinnutt, M. (2012) *Lecture Notes: Clinical Anaesthesia*. Chichester: Wiley-Blackwell.

4 Driscoll, P., Brown, T., Gwinnutt, C., Wardle, T. (1997) *A Simple Guide to Blood Gas Analysis*. London: BMJ Publishing Group.

5 O'Driscoll, B.R., Howard, L.S., Davidson, A.G. (2008) Guidelines for emergency oxygen use in adult patients. Thorax; 63(Suppl VI): vi1–73.

6 Martin, D.S., Grocott, M.P.W. (2013) Oxygen therapy in anaesthesia: the yin and yang of O_2. Br J Anaesth; 111: 867–71.

7 Weingart, S.D., Levitan, R.M. (2012) Preoxygenation and prevention of desaturation during emergency airway management. Ann Emerg Med; 59: 165–75.

Chapter

3

Basic airway management

Stephen Bush and David Ray

Objectives

The objectives of this chapter are to:

- Understand the importance of basic airway management in relation to advanced airway skills.
- Be familiar with basic airway management techniques.

Introduction

Basic airway management is the foundation for advanced airway skills.

Basic airway manoeuvres, although apparently simple, may be both difficult and life-saving. Basic airway management is a vital component of any airway intervention; there is little point acquiring expertise in advanced techniques if the practitioner cannot open the airway and ventilate the patient's lungs.

Airway obstruction can occur at any level from the mouth to the carina. Posterior tongue displacement, blood, secretions, teeth, vomit and foreign bodies are common causes. Oedema and direct airway injury are comparatively rare causes of airway obstruction. In most patients, a combination of positioning, airway manoeuvres, adjuncts and assisted ventilation will enable sufficient oxygenation to maintain life. These interventions are considered below.

Positioning

To optimize air flow, the head, neck and torso must be positioned to align the oral, pharyngeal and laryngeal axes. Figure 3.1 shows the C-shaped alignment

Emergency Airway Management, Second Edition, ed. Andrew Burtenshaw, Jonathan Benger and Jerry Nolan. Published by Cambridge University Press. © College of Emergency Medicine, London, 2015.

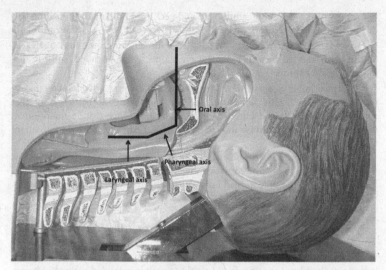

Figure 3.1 The C-shaped curve that is formed between the oral axis, pharyngeal axis and laryngeal axis when the head and neck are in the neutral position.

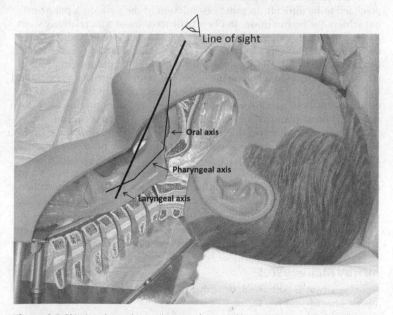

Figure 3.2 Aligning the oral axis, pharyngeal axis and laryngeal axis by flexing the neck and extending the head.

of the airway axes when the adult head and neck are in the neutral position. In this position the practitioner's view of the airway and larynx is not optimal.

In an adult the airway axes are aligned optimally when the neck is flexed on the torso and the head is extended on the neck, the so-called 'sniffing the morning air' position (Figure 3.2).

This position is easily achieved by placing a pillow or folded blanket under the patient's head. This flexes the neck on the torso, the thickness of the support determining the amount of neck flexion. Once this is maintained satisfactorily, the practitioner may gently extend the head on the neck to align the three airway axes.

Do not force the head and neck into this position in elderly patients or those with kyphosis or limited neck movement. Instead, support the patient's head and neck using pillows and bolsters to achieve the best possible position without using unnecessary force.

If a cervical spine injury is suspected, maintain the neck in a neutral position.

The most frequent positioning error is hyperextension of both the head and the neck; if head support is not used the neck is extended instead of being flexed, which can occlude the airway.

Positioning of the patient is even more important if the airway is predicted to be difficult. In some cases flexion of the neck on a pillow may not achieve the best position. In obese patients or those with relatively short necks, standard neck positioning may flex the head, forcing the chin onto the chest wall. This impedes access to the neck and may prevent the laryngoscope blade from entering the mouth because the anterior chest wall or the hand of an assistant applying cricoid pressure obstructs the handle. It also angles the oral axis forward. The key to correct positioning of the obese patient is to make sure that the external auditory meatus is on the same horizontal plane as the sternal notch. This can often be achieved by using a commercially available head-elevating laryngoscopy pillow or by placing one pillow under the shoulders and raising the head further using additional pillows. See Chapter 6 for further discussion. Raising the head-end of the trolley or bed also improves pre-oxygenation in obese patients by reducing the pressure of the abdominal contents on the diaphragm, thereby increasing the functional residual capacity. Optimal positioning is often best determined from the side rather than from the head of the patient.

These principles of positioning apply equally to basic airway interventions and to the more advanced airway skills of laryngoscopy and tracheal intubation.

Airway manoeuvres

Once the airway is positioned, two other movements may further improve the airway: chin lift and jaw thrust.

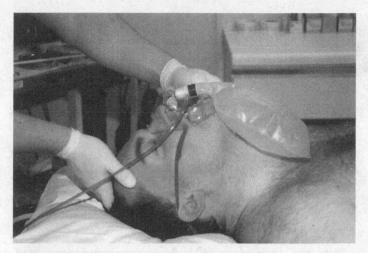

Figure 3.3 Chin lift.

Chin lift

Chin lift opens the airway by pulling the mandible forward and lifting the tongue off the posterior pharyngeal wall. The practitioner places the fingers of one hand under the mandible and lifts gently upwards (Figure 3.3). The thumb of the same hand can be used to depress the lower lip, thereby opening the mouth. The chin lift cannot be used easily at the same time as holding a facemask over the patient's face, as the practitioner's thumb obstructs the correct positioning of the facemask. It may also become uncomfortable for the practitioner to maintain this manoeuvre for a long time.

Jaw thrust

The jaw thrust manoeuvre enables the simultaneous application of a facemask. In this technique, the practitioner's fingers are placed under and behind the angles of the mandible. The thumbs may be placed as for the chin lift, to open the mouth, or used together with the index fingers to hold a mask onto the patient's face. The mandible is then lifted forwards and upwards, lifting the tongue off the posterior pharyngeal wall (Figure 3.4).

If these manoeuvres improve the airway significantly then better oxygenation may improve the patient's conscious level.

Suction

Suction is essential for removing any liquid in the upper airway. The sucker is not used as a diagnostic tool to see if liquid is present; it must be used gently,

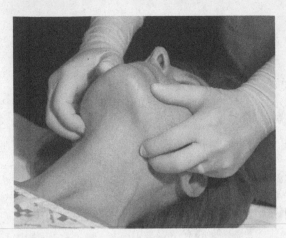

Figure 3.4 Jaw thrust. Courtesy of Mike Scott.

under direct vision. Advancing the tip blindly may cause airway trauma, vagal stimulation, increased intracranial pressure and vomiting. To avoid mucosal occlusion of the sucker tip use an intermediate negative pressure setting initially, and then adjust as required.

Airway adjuncts

If a manual manoeuvre is needed to open the airway an adjunct such as an oropharyngeal or nasopharyngeal airway will often enhance both ventilation and practitioner comfort, particularly if assisted ventilation is not required immediately, and the practitioner is not required to hold the facemask firmly on the patient's face. These devices enable the airway to be supported without the need for application of force by the practitioner.

Furthermore, in the presence of partial airway obstruction, the volume of gas expelled passively on expiration may be less than that introduced during positive pressure ventilation, resulting in a progressive increase in intrathoracic pressure. Higher inspiratory pressure is required to produce adequate ventilation for subsequent breaths, promoting gastric inflation, diaphragmatic splinting and aspiration risk. The use of an airway adjunct early can aid effective exhalation, thereby preventing this cycle.

Oropharyngeal airways

Oropharyngeal airways are hard plastic devices that are shaped to follow the contours of the oropharynx (Figure 3.5). They have a lumen to maintain airway patency and enable passage of a suction catheter to clear the oropharynx. Their shape lifts the tongue off the posterior pharyngeal wall, and the wide lumen presents little resistance to air flow.

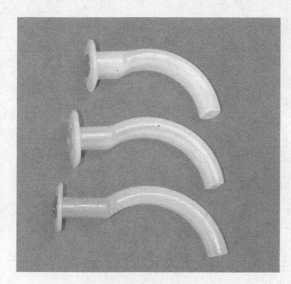

Figure 3.5
Oropharyngeal
airways.

Indications: The primary indication for oropharyngeal airway insertion is an obstructed airway, or an airway that requires active manoeuvres for maintenance of airway patency. These devices should be used only in patients with obtunded cough and gag reflexes (see below).

Sizing: The airway is sized by placing it on the patient's face and measuring its length along a vertical line from the patient's incisors to the angle of the jaw. Correct sizing is important to reduce the likelihood of obstruction.

Insertion: The airway is inserted upside down into the mouth. Once the tip has passed the hard palate the airway is rotated 180 degrees and advanced over the tongue. An alternative method is to use a tongue depressor or a laryngoscope blade to depress the tongue and then insert the airway the correct way up under direct vision.

Complications: Insertion of an oropharyngeal airway in a patient who retains some airway reflexes may cause gagging, laryngospasm, vomiting, raised intracranial pressure and predispose to aspiration of gastric or oropharyngeal contents.

Limitations: As a general guide, a patient who tolerates an oropharyngeal airway has impaired airway protective reflexes indicating the need for placement of a definitive airway. The oropharyngeal airway maintains, but does not protect, the airway; however, it will enable oxygenation before tracheal intubation. Should the increase in oxygenation improve the conscious level then intubation may not be necessary. If this occurs, or if the patient's conscious level improves for any other reason, the oral airway may need to be removed.

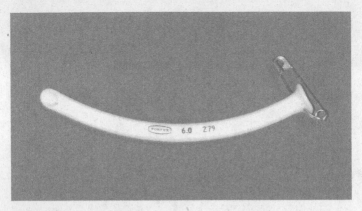

Figure 3.6 Nasopharyngeal airway.

A patient requiring an oral airway must not be left unattended.

Nasopharyngeal airways

Nasopharyngeal airways are soft, curved tubes with a bevel at one end and a flange at the other (Figure 3.6). Some airways are supplied with safety pins to avoid displacement into the nostril: the safety pin is placed through the flange of the device before the airway is inserted.

Indications: Nasopharyngeal airways improve the airway by splinting open the posterior nasopharynx. Their great advantage over oropharyngeal airways is that they may be inserted in patients with intact airway reflexes without the significant risk of gagging, vomiting or aspiration associated with oral devices. They are also very useful in patients with limited mouth opening.

Sizing: The traditional methods for sizing a nasopharyngeal airway (measurement against the patient's little finger or anterior nares) do not correlate with airway anatomy, and are unreliable. An appropriate size of nasopharyngeal airway in adults is 6 mm internal diameter for an average female and 7 mm internal diameter for an average male. If the airway is too long it may stimulate airway reflexes and induce vomiting. If too short, the tip may become occluded by the nasal mucosa.

Insertion: The technique of insertion is simple and must be gentle. Select the nostril that appears larger and less obstructed by the nasal septum. Lubricate the device and the nostril with a water-based gel. The tip of the airway is inserted into the nostril and directed posteriorly along the transverse floor of the nose. Slight rotation of the airway during insertion may be helpful.

If insertion of a nasopharyngeal airway into a nostril is difficult, it is usually easier (and safer) to use the other nostril.

Some resistance is often felt as the airway passes the turbinates; if this is significant use a smaller airway so that complications are minimized. Insertion of a second airway into the other nostril may improve air flow.

Complications: Nasopharyngeal airways may cause profuse haemorrhage; use of a vasoconstrictor spray before insertion may reduce the risk of bleeding.

Limitations: Relative contra-indications to nasopharyngeal airway insertion include basal skull fracture or significant facial injury with damage to the cribriform plate. The presence of these injuries may result in intracranial placement of the airway; however, this complication is unlikely and in the presence of life-threatening hypoxaemia and where insertion of an oropharyngeal airway is not possible, gentle and careful insertion of a nasopharyngeal airway using the above technique may be life-saving.

The effectiveness of any airway manoeuvre or adjunct must always be assessed after it has been completed.

Oxygenation

Spontaneous ventilation

Methods of oxygen delivery to a spontaneously breathing patient are described in Chapter 2.

Assisted ventilation

Even if spontaneous ventilatory efforts are present, they may be inadequate for effective gas exchange. Examine the chest to assess the breathing rate and tidal volume. Arterial blood gas analysis is helpful in determining whether assisted ventilation is needed.

Should assisted ventilation be needed, the usual first step is a bag-mask technique. Although apparently simple, effective bag-mask ventilation requires several potentially difficult manoeuvres to be performed well.

Mask application: The correct size of mask must be used. This is one that covers the face from the nasal bridge to the alveolar ridge. Transparent masks are recommended to enable observation of the inner surface for 'fogging' or vomiting. Some slight movement of the mask on the face is usually required for an optimal seal. Hold the mask on the face with the thumb and index finger after gently opening the airway. Spread the other fingers out along the lower border of the mandible and, ideally, place the little finger behind the angle of the mandible. These three fingers should pull the mandible up to the mask, rather than the mask being pushed down onto the mandible. Insertion of an oropharyngeal and/or nasopharyngeal airway may assist in maintaining the airway. In the unconscious or obtunded patient the jaw thrust manoeuvre is very useful when used in conjunction with an airway adjunct and application of the facemask.

Sealing techniques: A poor mask seal may occur if the patient has a beard, is edentulous or is emaciated. The use of a water-based gel, leaving well-fitting dentures in place, or packing the cheeks with gauze rolls may improve the seal. A poor seal will lead to an air leak and cause poor ventilation.

Choice of equipment: Most practitioners are familiar with the self-inflating bag. This device comprises a thick-walled ventilation bag, a reservoir, and a one-way valve that prevents subsequent inspiration of expired gas. The valve mechanism can become stuck if blocked by secretions, blood or vomit. Most self-inflating bags are now single use only, but if a reusable bag is used a breathing filter is attached before use. The self-inflating bag re-expands after compression even without gas flow, and therefore enables ventilation to continue in the event of a gas supply failure. For this reason a self-inflating bag-mask must accompany patients who require, or may require, assisted ventilation during all transfers. Remember to check that the oxygen supply is connected and turned on – a self-inflating bag will still inflate in the absence of oxygen.

Although the self-inflating bag is an excellent device for assisted ventilation, the one-way valve causes some resistance to gas flow in spontaneous ventilation. If the patient is breathing adequately, supplemental oxygen is best provided by other means (see Chapter 2).

> A self-inflating bag-mask must accompany the transfer of any patient who may require assisted ventilation.

Ventilation: Effective assisted ventilation requires a good mask seal to minimize leakage. Avoid high airway pressures; this reduces the possibility of gastric inflation, with subsequent regurgitation and aspiration. Cricoid pressure may be applied to reduce this risk, but is difficult to maintain for a long time. Partial airway obstruction can cause high airway pressures; therefore a two-person technique is recommended, especially for inexperienced practitioners. This technique enables one practitioner to use both hands to open the airway and hold the mask firmly on the face whilst a second practitioner compresses the bag. The practitioner opening the airway has both hands available for the task, and is likely to be much more effective.

If the airway pressure remains high while using the two-person technique, consider insertion of an airway adjunct. If necessary, insertion of a nasopharyngeal airway into each nostril along with an oropharyngeal airway may be helpful. Use suction to remove any foreign material in the airway, and ensure the patient is correctly positioned.

> The first solution for failed bag-mask ventilation is better bag-mask ventilation!

If the patient is making some respiratory effort, synchronize assisted ventilations with the patient's own efforts. Poor synchronization will cause high airway pressures, inadequate ventilation and subsequent gastric inflation with potential aspiration.

Summary

- Basic airway management is the foundation of advanced airway skills.
- Correct positioning of the head and neck is essential to ensure the best airway, but be careful if a cervical spine injury is suspected, or if the patient is elderly or kyphotic.
- In obese patients ensure that the chin is higher than the highest point of the chest or abdomen.
- Airway manoeuvres may also be needed to open the airway.
- Airway adjuncts such as oro- and nasopharyngeal airways are useful in supporting the airway.
- Synchronized assisted ventilation is required when respiratory efforts are inadequate; this may be achieved with a bag-mask or anaesthetic breathing system.

Further reading

1 Marx, J., Hockberger, R., Walls, R. (2013) *Rosen's Emergency Medicine: Concepts and Clinical Practice*, 8th edn. Philadelphia: Elsevier.

2 Healy, T., Knight, P.R.(2003) *Wylie & Churchill-Davidson's A Practice of Anesthesia*, 7th edn. London: Arnold.

3 Walls, R.M., Murphy, M.F.. (2012) *Manual of Emergency Airway Management*, 4th edn. Philadelphia: Lippincott, Williams & Wilkins.

4 Brasel, K., Kortbeek, J.B., Turki S.A. *et al.* (2012) *Advanced Trauma Life Support Course Provider Manual*, 9th edn. Chicago: American College of Surgeons.

5 Nolan, J., Soar, J., Lockey, A. *et al.* (2011) *Advanced Life Support*, 6th edn. London: Resuscitation Council (UK).

6 Roberts, K., Whalley, H., Bleetman, A. (2005) The nasopharyngeal airway: dispelling myths and establishing the facts. Emerg Med J; 22: 394–6.

Indications for intubation

Colin A. Graham and Dermot McKeown

Objectives

The objectives of this chapter are to:

- Understand that all airway care starts with basic manoeuvres and oxygen.
- Recognize four situations in which intubation is likely to be required.
- Be able to distinguish between an immediate need for intubation and an urgent need for intubation.
- Be aware of important reversible causes of an impaired airway or ventilation.

Introduction

Control of the airway is control of the clinical situation. Early effective airway care can establish a safe position from which all other priorities flow; conversely, misjudged airway decisions can make a bad situation worse. It is therefore crucial that the practitioner managing the airway formulates a clear plan, communicates this to the team, and calls for help when appropriate.

The decision to intubate or not is often the key first decision in treating a critically ill or injured patient. Tracheal intubation with a cuffed tube secures the airway and enables oxygenation and ventilation of the lungs. It protects the lungs from aspiration of blood or vomit and enables sedation to be given safely without risk of respiratory compromise.

However, the procedure can be technically difficult and failed intubation or a misplaced tracheal tube can be rapidly lethal. The injection of drugs to achieve intubation also carries a further set of pharmacological complications, and commits the patient to ventilatory support.

Emergency Airway Management, Second Edition, ed. Andrew Burtenshaw, Jonathan Benger and Jerry Nolan. Published by Cambridge University Press. © College of Emergency Medicine, London, 2015.

Intubation is indicated when the risks of continuing with basic airway support are greater than the risks of intubation.

Basic airway manoeuvres always form the mainstay of the immediate management of the emergency airway, however briefly applied.

General considerations

There are four clinical situations in which intubation may be indicated:
1. Apnoeic patient.
2. Patient with an obstructed/partially obstructed airway where basic airway care is ineffective.
3. Patient requiring invasive respiratory support for oxygenation or ventilatory failure.
4. Patient in whom basic airway care is effective, but whose predicted clinical course includes a high probability of airway obstruction, aspiration or ventilatory failure.

Within these groups there is often considerable overlap, and several indications may coexist. The urgency of the intubation must be decided for each patient. Broadly, there are:

• *Immediate intubations,* in which the patient is deteriorating rapidly and definitive airway care is required with a minimum of delay.
• *Urgent intubations,* in which basic techniques can maintain the physiology of the patient for a short period, pending intubation.
• *Observant situations,* in which no indication for intubation currently exists, and the patient can be observed closely for any deterioration.

The initial step of providing supplemental oxygen and basic airway care must never be overlooked.

The success of supplemental oxygen and basic airway manoeuvres is critical in deciding both the need for and the urgency of the intubation. For example, a patient in coma with obstruction of an anatomically normal airway can usually be oxygenated effectively for a short period using basic techniques with or without bag-mask support. Urgent intubation may then follow to prevent respiratory failure and aspiration. Conversely, a patient in coma with facial injuries or vomit in the airway who cannot be adequately oxygenated using basic techniques requires immediate intubation to avoid severe hypoxaemia.

It is also important to carry out an early rapid assessment of the likely technical difficulty of intubation (see Chapter 5). If there is a high risk of failed intubation, then this must be balanced against the assessed urgency of the situation. For example, a patient with partial airway obstruction from a laryngeal malignancy who is well oxygenated is likely to be technically difficult to intubate and can wait for expert assessment and specialist techniques. Conversely, a patient with partial airway obstruction from burns who is hypoxaemic is also likely to be technically difficult to intubate, but requires immediate placement of a definitive airway by the first practitioner with the appropriate skills.

Airway decision-making must not be dissociated from the clinical situation. In some cases, there may be reversible causes for airway obstruction, respiratory compromise or a reduced conscious level. If these are identified, they are treated while continuing basic airway care. Clearly, if such measures are not rapidly effective, it may be necessary to proceed to definitive airway management. Reversible causes are specified in each of the following sections.

Take special care in patients with a tracheostomy who present with airway obstruction or respiratory distress. The default action in this situation is to clear both the upper airway and the tracheostomy, and apply oxygen to both the face and the stoma simultaneously. Further assessment to determine if the tracheostomy is an end tracheostomy (i.e. the patient has had a laryngectomy) or if the patient has a patent or potentially patent upper airway is urgently required.

If the patient has had a laryngectomy, conventional intubation is not possible and rapid sequence induction (RSI) should not be attempted. In these patients, passing a tracheal tube or tracheostomy tube into the stoma may be necessary to control the airway and provide controlled ventilation. Summon senior help early if a patient with a tracheostomy presents with an airway emergency. Detailed guidelines for the management of the airway in patients with tracheostomies are available from the National Tracheostomy Safety Project (see Further reading).

Intubation may not always be appropriate for patients with end-stage diseases. If in doubt, treat, but where time permits obtain further information.

Table 4.1 Reversible causes of airway obstruction or respiratory compromise

- Arrhythmia (e.g. ventricular fibrillation)
- Fitting
- Rapidly reversible causes of coma, including hypoglycaemia and opioid overdose
- Bronchospasm
- Pneumothorax
- Acute pulmonary oedema
- Anaphylaxis

Clinical indications for intubation

Apnoeic patient

These patients are deeply unconscious with no significant respiratory effort, and are often in full cardiorespiratory arrest. Basic airway manoeuvres are instituted and bag-mask ventilation commenced with supplemental high-flow oxygen. Advanced life support protocols are followed.

At a suitable point during resuscitation the patient should be intubated; however, the place of intubation in cardiopulmonary resuscitation has been de-emphasized and it should be performed only by a skilled operator who is able to complete the procedure with a very short (<10 s) interruption in chest compressions. Intubation does enable more effective ventilation and oxygenation, frees up team members from holding the facemask, and prevents further aspiration secondary to distension of the stomach from bag-mask ventilation.

As the patient is profoundly unconscious, attempts at intubation can be carried out without the assistance of induction or neuromuscular blocking drugs. The airway reflexes are absent, there is no autonomic response to airway manipulation and the vocal cords are open. Use waveform capnography to confirm the position of the tracheal tube and to assist in the recognition of a return of spontaneous circulation. Even during cardiac arrest, a correctly placed tracheal tube will lead to a typical, but attenuated, capnography waveform whilst CPR is ongoing. If skilled personnel or capnography are not available, a supraglottic airway device is preferable.

Reversible cause: ventricular fibrillation. Attempts at restoring a spontaneous circulation take priority over intubation (but not basic airway care). If output is quickly restored by defibrillation, with a rapid return to consciousness, intubation is not usually required.

Patient with obstructed or partially obstructed airway who does not respond to basic airway manoeuvres

There are groups of patients for whom basic airway techniques are relatively ineffective, and they may require immediate definitive airway placement. These patients are uncommon – not because airway obstruction is uncommon, but because almost all patients can be helped by high-quality basic airway care.

Patients may fall into the immediate category because of:

- anatomical disruption of their airway;
- active aspiration of blood or vomit.

These situations are often complicated by reduced conscious level because of hypoxaemia from the obstructed airway, or other coexisting mechanisms (e.g. head injury, overdose). The particular problem with this group is that not only are these patients in need of prompt intubation to prevent hypoxic brain injury, but they can also be technically demanding to intubate. The recognition of such a patient, or prior warning of the arrival of such a patient, should prompt an early call for senior assistance.

Likely clinical scenarios include:

Facial trauma

Disruption to normal facial anatomy may render an airway unmaintainable without intubation. This is particularly true of complex midface fractures, where the upper airway is compromised by the displaced bony segment, and of complex jaw fractures, where the tongue loses its normal support and falls back to obstruct the airway.

It may also be impossible to maintain the airway in facial trauma because of severe haemorrhage from facial bones and soft tissues. The patient may be inhaling blood or exsanguinating from blood loss. Packing to stop the bleeding may further compromise the airway.

Patients with complex facial injuries often also have head injuries, rendering them combative or comatose with impaired protective airway reflexes.

> The finding of a hypoxaemic, obtunded trauma patient with severe facial injuries and a compromised airway necessitates an early decision to intubate.

While preparations are made, basic airway care and supplemental oxygen are provided. These situations are technically challenging and have a very high potential for failed intubation. Call for senior assistance immediately. Preparations are made for a failed intubation – or rapid conversion to a surgical airway ('plan B').

Laryngeal disruption/swelling

Direct injury to the larynx may make the airway impossible to maintain. Blunt trauma to the front of the neck may fracture the larynx and produce stridor, crepitus and surgical emphysema.

Similarly, a penetrating injury to the neck may produce an expanding haematoma that compresses and distorts the airway, causing stridor, hoarseness and respiratory distress.

Infection, anaphylaxis, radiotherapy or burns may cause internal swelling of the larynx or epiglottis. As with external damage to the larynx, this may produce hoarseness, stridor and respiratory distress.

In all these situations, the airway is compromised and likely to deteriorate quickly to full obstruction. Stridor in an adult is a particularly worrying sign. Simple airway manoeuvres will not be effective, although supplemental oxygen can buy some time before hypoxaemia occurs.

This situation is very hazardous, as the distortion of normal anatomy can make intubation extremely difficult, or impossible. Furthermore, a rescue surgical airway via cricothyroidotomy may also be technically difficult. Summon senior anaesthetic assistance immediately, along with a surgeon capable of performing emergency tracheostomy.

Despite the risks, once the patient begins to become hypoxaemic, intubation must be attempted urgently by the most experienced person present before the patient becomes impossible to intubate. If adequate oxygenation can be achieved using supplemental oxygen, sitting posture and suction, it is safer to defer airway intervention until senior anaesthetic assistance arrives. The balance of risk in these difficult cases depends on the experience and airway skills of the most senior doctor present.

Coma with difficult airway or profuse vomiting

Patients may have reduced conscious level through head injury, cerebral haemorrhage, metabolic coma or drug overdose. The airway can usually be maintained for a short period using simple airway techniques, while preparations for intubation are made. The provision of a definitive airway is therefore urgent, rather than immediate.

In some circumstances, however, this is not possible and the airway is unmaintainable, even if anatomically normal. It is important to distinguish these patients as they may require immediate intubation to prevent severe hypoxaemia.

Conditions causing difficulty in maintaining airway in coma may include:

- prolonged seizures;
- pre-existing characteristics (limited neck movement, facial hair, obesity);
- active aspiration (vomit or blood in the upper airway).

All these patients may also be difficult to intubate, and this should be taken into account when deciding on the timing of airway management.

The common clinical feature to all of these situations is a patient who has an airway that is compromised by fluid (blood, vomit) and/or anatomical disruption. This will manifest as noisy breathing, usually with snoring, gurgling or stridor, and will be associated with marked respiratory distress unless or until the conscious level decreases. Later, hypoventilation occurs with reduced air entry progressing to apnoea with weak, tugging respiratory efforts. Hypoxaemia can be a relatively late sign, especially if the patient is receiving supplemental oxygen, and because the pulse oximeter cannot detect retention of CO_2.

The management of all such patients consists of basic airway care, suction and high-flow oxygen. The response to these initial actions will determine the urgency of proceeding to intubation, coupled with an assessment of the likely technical difficulty in carrying out the procedure.

Reversible causes: fitting, coma and anaphylaxis

Even in some very difficult to maintain airways, there may be reversible causes that should be sought, since their presence changes the clinical situation, and in some cases may even avoid the need for intubation. Treat convulsions with intravenous benzodiazepines. Treat coma caused by hypotension, hypoglycaemia or opioid overdose with appropriate measures. Laryngeal oedema from anaphylaxis may respond to parenteral adrenaline, and laryngeal obstruction caused by haemorrhage within the neck can be relieved in some cases, e.g. after thyroid surgery by opening the surgical wound.

Patient requiring invasive respiratory support for ventilatory failure or critical oxygenation

Patients may require a definitive airway to enable invasive ventilation for respiratory failure. There are two overlapping physiological types of respiratory failure.

Type 1 respiratory failure

Failure of oxygenation with no CO_2 retention caused by conditions such as:

- severe chest trauma;
- pneumonia;
- acute respiratory distress syndrome;
- acute pulmonary oedema.

In these cases, there is usually severe $\dot{V}/\dot{Q}$ mismatching. A decision to proceed to intubation is usually taken after attempts at oxygenation by non-invasive means have failed. The amount of respiratory effort made by the patient will often determine the urgency with which respiratory support is instituted. It is preferable to intubate the patient before exhaustion or type 2 respiratory failure supervenes.

Type 2 respiratory failure

Failure of ventilation with CO_2 retention caused by conditions such as:

- chronic obstructive pulmonary disease/asthma;
- coma/overdose;
- neuromuscular disorders.

In these cases hypoventilation with slow or inadequate respiration predominates; oxygenation may be adequate. In mild cases in conscious patients who can cooperate, non-invasive ventilation may be appropriate, but if the conscious level is impaired or the patient becomes severely acidaemic, invasive ventilation is required. In severe cases, the patient may require bag-mask ventilation to maintain adequate gas exchange pending institution of formal ventilatory support.

It is not possible to deliver more than 80% oxygen via a facemask with a reservoir, and ventilation of obtunded patients by non-invasive means (including bag-mask) carries a high aspiration risk because of gaseous distension of the stomach.

In all these patients, there is usually some time to optimize conditions and fully prepare before intubation. The intubation of patients who are hypoxaemic and/or acidaemic carries a significant risk of complications.

Reversible causes: bronchospasm, pneumothorax, acute pulmonary oedema and opioids

Seek potentially reversible causes of respiratory failure and treat while basic support is carried out. Specifically, treat bronchospasm with bronchodilators, pneumothorax with chest drainage, pulmonary oedema with diuretics and nitrates (not opioids in respiratory failure) and where possible, reverse respiratory depressants (e.g. opioids, neuromuscular blocking drugs).

Patients in whom basic airway care is effective, but the predicted clinical course includes high probability of airway obstruction, aspiration or ventilatory failure

Many critically ill patients require intubation because there is a significant risk of adverse events developing. The urgency with which this is required will depend on the predicted clinical course for that patient.

The patients to whom this applies are those with a significant risk of:

- respiratory arrest;
- airway obstruction;
- aspiration;
- respiratory failure.

Consider the patient environment. There is a greater risk for patients in circumstances where airway interventions cannot be achieved easily, e.g. during transport or CT scanning.

> If the patient has an airway that could become compromised, intubate before transport or scanning.

This group includes those patients who require basic airway manoeuvres (e.g. an oropharyngeal airway) to maintain a satisfactory airway. Commonly, they are unconscious patients who have impaired airway protective reflexes with a high risk of aspiration and respiratory depression. It also includes patients who need sedation in whom there is a high risk of respiratory failure.

Likely clinical situations include the following:

Potentially compromised airway anatomy: burns, laryngeal tumour, epiglottitis, anaphylaxis. Patients with distortion of their airway caused by malignancy, trauma or infection may present with signs of established airway obstruction; however, they may also present earlier with signs of an airway at risk.

Common examples include:

- neck swelling with penetrating trauma;
- hoarseness with facial burns;
- tongue swelling caused by anaphylaxis or angio-oedema (common causes of angio-oedema include non-steroidal anti-inflammatory drugs and ACE inhibitors).

Often, the arterial blood is well oxygenated and patients can cope, as long as they are in the sitting position and given supplemental oxygen. The clinical context must be taken into account. If the airway is likely to deteriorate rapidly, e.g. because of burns or an expanding haematoma, intubate the patient's trachea as soon as possible. If the patient is likely to improve rapidly with treatment, such as in anaphylaxis or angio-oedema, then intubation may be replaced with careful observation and immediate effective treatment.

If a patient develops complete airway obstruction and worsening hypoxaemia, call for senior assistance and intubate immediately using standard RSI techniques.

Head injury/coma. Conditions causing reduced consciousness with a particular risk of airway or ventilatory compromise:

- head injury;
- intracranial haemorrhage;
- overdose (particularly tricyclic antidepressants);
- prolonged seizures;
- hepatic encephalopathy.

In the presence of head injury or raised intracranial pressure (ICP), hypoventilation and hypercapnia increases cerebral oedema. In these patients airway and ventilatory complications frequently occur during transport to other hospitals or clinical areas such as the CT scanner.

Patients with a Glasgow Coma Scale (GCS) score of 8 or less are at high risk of aspiration because of loss of airway reflexes. They also frequently have abnormalities of respiratory drive with a tendency to hypoventilation and respiratory arrest.

Treatment of these patients starts with basic airway manoeuvres and supplemental oxygen. If the airway cannot be maintained, immediate intubation is required. Otherwise, if it is clear that there are no immediately reversible causes for the coma, make preparations for intubation. Ensure the patient is pre-oxygenated adequately and positioned optimally. Hypotension is also potentially harmful, particularly in head injury; optimize cardiovascular stability as much as possible before and during intubation (see 'Trauma and raised intracranial pressure' in Chapter 11.2 for further information).

Impaired consciousness with agitation

Patients with a GCS score of 9–12 may need to be intubated, even if there is no airway obstruction and no ventilatory failure. Obtunded, agitated patients, particularly those who have suffered multiple injuries, including head injuries, can be exceptionally difficult to manage without anaesthesia. This is because procedures such as CT scanning become impossible, and placing lines and tubes hazardous; furthermore, many of these patients will deteriorate and are at risk of developing airway obstruction, hypoventilation and aspiration.

In this group, it is essential to first seek reversible causes of agitation, such as pain, shock, hypoglycaemia or a full bladder. If these are not present and the predicted clinical course is that the patient is likely to remain unmanageable, then consider RSI and intubation. This is particularly the case for highly agitated head-injured patients, who are at risk of becoming comatose with very little warning.

Intubating an uncooperative patient also carries considerable risks. Inadequate pre-oxygenation, loss of venous access and suboptimal positioning are all potential factors that may contribute to intubation difficulty. In some cases, sedation may be required to control the situation before undertaking a formal RSI. This is discussed further in Chapter 8.

Severe shock with acidaemia

Some critically ill patients with septic shock can develop intractable acidosis and impaired consciousness, which necessitates ventilatory support. Attempts at improving the shock state with supplemental oxygen, fluid resuscitation and inotropes form the mainstay of initial management. However, if it is clear that the patient's clinical course is deteriorating, consider intubation to optimize oxygenation, remove the work of breathing and assist in the correction of metabolic acidosis. Patients who have been compensating for a lactic acidosis with a high minute volume before intubation will require a high minute volume after intubation, otherwise their acidaemia will worsen and may result in cardiovascular collapse.

Careful choice of induction drug and dose is essential to avoid severe hypotension. If possible, intubate these patients with invasive arterial monitoring already established, and with the involvement of experienced intensive care staff.

The feature common to all of these patients is that on initial assessment they either do not require, or improve significantly with, basic airway manoeuvres and supplemental oxygen. Although this implies that the need for intubation is not immediate, they may still be candidates for emergency intubation. Patients may deteriorate quickly, e.g. a burns patient may develop stridor and hypoxaemia, a head-injured patient may fit or vomit, and a septic patient may develop severe respiratory distress.

These events upgrade the clinical situation to an immediate need for intubation. However, as many of these situations are accompanied by considerable intubation risks, an investment of time in organizing experienced personnel and suitable equipment, together with adequate preparation of the patient, are both possible and desirable.

Reversible causes: hypoglycaemia and fitting

Some patients with impaired conscious level are likely to have a benign clinical course, such as those who are hypoglycaemic or post-ictal. These patients do not require intubation unless they do not respond rapidly to treatment.

Summary

- Intubation is indicated when the risks of continuing basic airway support exceed the risks of intubation and there are no rapidly reversible factors.
- Intubation is always preceded by basic airway care and supplemental oxygen.
- Immediate intubation is required if basic techniques cannot provide adequate oxygenation.

Acknowledgement

This chapter has been updated from the first edition chapter, which was written by Tim Parke, Dermot McKeown and Colin Graham.

Further reading

1   Resuscitation Council. Advanced life support guidelines. Available at: http://www.resus.org.uk/pages/als.pdf (accessed November 2014).

2   Trauma.Org. Airway management of the trauma victim. Available at: http://www.trauma.org/index.php/main/article/377/ (accessed November 2014).

3   Royal College of Physicians of London. Non-invasive ventilation guidelines. Available at: http://www.rcplondon.ac.uk/resources/concise-guidelines-non-invasive-ventilation-chronic-obstructive-pulmonary-disease (accessed November 2014).

4   The National Tracheostomy Safety Project (NTSP). Available at: http://www.tracheostomy.org.uk (accessed July 2014).

Chapter

5

Airway assessment

Dominic Williamson and Jerry Nolan

Objectives

The objectives of this chapter are to:

- Discuss the rationale for airway assessment.
- Outline a pre-anaesthetic patient assessment.
- Evaluate methods of airway assessment.
- Identify patients who may be difficult to ventilate and/or intubate.
- Identify patients that may require a different airway intervention.

Introduction

During elective anaesthesia a failed airway ('cannot intubate, cannot oxygenate') occurs in 0.01–0.03% of cases. Difficult intubation, defined as the need for more than three attempts, occurs in 1.15–3.8% of elective surgical cases, and is usually related to a poor view at laryngoscopy. However, the characteristics of patients requiring intubation or assisted ventilation outside the operating room are different to those undergoing elective surgical procedures, and the incidence of difficult intubation is significantly higher in emergency departments, as demonstrated by the Royal College of Anaesthetists' Fourth National Audit Project (NAP4). More importantly, a failed airway may occur at least ten times more frequently in the emergency setting; in the United States, 0.5% of intubations recorded in the National Emergency Airway Registry (NEAR) required a surgical airway. In a recent Scottish study, 57/671 (8.5%) of patients undergoing rapid sequence induction in the emergency department

Emergency Airway Management, Second Edition, ed. Andrew Burtenshaw, Jonathan Benger and Jerry Nolan. Published by Cambridge University Press. © College of Emergency Medicine, London, 2015.

had Cormack and Lehane grade 3 or 4 views at laryngoscopy (see below), and two (0.3%) required a surgical airway.

Given these data, difficulties with the airway must be expected in all emergency patients, and appropriate preparation undertaken. Some features may indicate a particularly high likelihood of airway difficulties, and in these cases modification of practice may reduce complications and improve outcome.

Definition of a difficult airway

A difficult airway is categorized by:

Difficult mask ventilation. Difficult mask ventilation occurs when the patient's anatomy or injuries make it impossible to maintain adequate ventilation and oxygenation with a facemask and simple airway adjuncts alone.

Difficult intubation. Difficult intubation is defined when an experienced laryngoscopist, using direct laryngoscopy, requires:

1. more than two attempts with the same blade or;
2. a change in the blade or an adjunct to a direct laryngoscope (e.g. bougie) or;
3. use of an alternative device or technique following failed intubation with direct laryngoscopy.

Difficult view at laryngoscopy. The view at direct laryngoscopy has been classified by Cormack and Lehane (Figure 5.1). A difficult view is defined as being unable to see any portion of the vocal cords with conventional laryngoscopy (Cormack and Lehane grades 3 and 4). These views are associated with more difficult or even impossible intubations under direct vision. Although this may not help at initial presentation, the grade of view at laryngoscopy must be recorded because it may influence the approach to future airway management by other healthcare professionals.

Grade 1 The vocal cords are visible
Grade 2 The vocals cords are only partly visible
Grade 3 Only the epiglottis is seen
Grade 4 The epiglottis cannot be seen

Difficult cricothyroidotomy. Failure to intubate the trachea combined with an inability to oxygenate the patient using a bag-mask or supraglottic airway device will necessitate a surgical airway. Occasionally, patient-specific features may render the cricothyroid membrane inaccessible. This makes induction of anaesthesia particularly risky because if the airway is lost it may be irretrievable, and oxygenating the patient will be impossible

Table 5.1 Pre-anaesthetic assessment of emergency patients where time allows

- Comprehensive history
- Cardiorespiratory status
- Conscious level
- Focal/global neurological signs
- Assessment of face and neck
- Assessment for pneumothorax
- Abdominal and pelvic assessment for surgical signs
- Body morphology

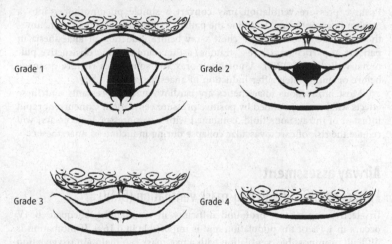

Grade 1   Grade 2

Grade 3   Grade 4

Figure 5.1 The Cormack and Lehane classification of laryngeal view.

General assessment of patients before inducing anaesthesia

Few patients require immediate induction of anaesthesia and intubation. Some time is usually available for a clinical assessment and, where possible, a comprehensive evaluation of the patient is required before inducing anaesthesia (see Table 5.1).

When time allows, obtain a good history including current medication and allergies, previous medical and surgical problems, last oral intake, and details of the patient's current condition. If available, previous medical records can be invaluable. Patients and relatives may have been informed about any serious problems, including airway difficulties, occurring during previous anaesthetics. A MedicAlert bracelet system has been advocated for patients with difficult airways, and may be carried by some.

Document clearly the pre-anaesthetic findings and communicate them to the team responsible for the patient's continuing care.

Once a patient is anaesthetized some physical signs will be lost, e.g. abdominal guarding or abnormal neurology. Before inducing anaesthesia, pay attention to:

- the Glasgow Coma Scale (GCS);
- focal neurological signs;
- evidence of pathology in the chest, abdomen or pelvis.

Positive pressure ventilation may convert a simple pneumothorax into a tension pneumothorax. Examine the patient and look for signs of a pneumothorax. Consider obtaining a chest x-ray before induction of anaesthesia in patients at particular risk, e.g. trauma, asthma and chronic obstructive pulmonary disease (COPD). A pneumothorax will sometimes require drainage before or immediately after induction of anaesthesia.

Most intravenous anaesthetics are cardiovascular depressants and these effects will be compounded by positive pressure ventilation. Concurrent rapid infusion of intravenous fluid, combined with a vasopressor if necessary, will reduce the risk of cardiovascular collapse during induction of anaesthesia.

Airway assessment

Predicting difficulty in bag-mask ventilation (BMV)

In elective anaesthesia profound difficulty in maintaining adequate BMV occurs in 1.4% of the population and is impossible in 0.16%. If intubation is difficult or impossible, ventilation with a bag-mask can maintain oxygenation until the airway is secured. Difficulty with facemask ventilation is a serious problem, and every effort should be made to anticipate this complication. The combination of difficult mask ventilation and difficult laryngoscopy occurs in 0.4% of the general anaesthesia population. In many cases, difficulty with facemask ventilation may be resolved by use of simple airway manoeuvres, adjuncts or a change in technique. If these fail, insertion of a supraglottic airway device may enable oxygenation and ventilation until a definitive airway is established.

Difficult facemask ventilation will occur if it is not possible to establish a good seal, if airway patency is difficult to maintain, if airway resistance is high, or if lung and chest wall compliance is poor. A study of patients undergoing elective surgery identified five criteria that were independent predictors of difficult mask ventilation: age > 55 years, body mass index > 26 kg m^{-2}, beard, lack of teeth, and a history of snoring. Combinations of these factors significantly increase the likelihood of difficulties during BMV.

Features likely to cause difficulty in achieving a good seal with a facemask

- dysmorphic or asymmetrical facial features;
- a beard or moustache; this may be rectified by the application of petroleum jelly or aqueous lubricant, although the resulting slippery conditions may cause additional difficulty;
- significant cachexia, missing molar teeth or missing dentures causing sunken cheeks; where possible, leave well-fitting dentures in place; when this is not feasible, pad the cheeks out with dressing gauze, but ensure that all gauze is subsequently removed to avoid inadvertent airway occlusion following later extubation;
- facial trauma, particularly through and through cheek lacerations and unstable bony injuries.

Features likely to cause difficulty in maintaining an airway without intubation

- a short jaw or inability to bring bottom incisors in front of top incisors (prognath);
- immobilized neck;
- unstable facial bony injuries;
- upper airway obstruction, e.g. blood or vomit, retropharyngeal swelling such as haematoma or infection;
- obesity;
- macroglossia;
- history of snoring.

Features likely to make it difficult to ventilate the lungs

- abdominal distension/diaphragmatic splinting;
- lower airways obstruction, e.g. asthma, pneumothorax;
- obesity.

Predicting difficult intubation

Most tests used to predict difficult intubation have poor sensitivity and specificity, particularly in the emergency patient when it can be difficult to obtain a comprehensive evaluation. If a particular feature associated with difficult intubation is present, whilst more likely, it does not necessarily mean that the patient will be difficult to intubate. Likewise if a feature is absent it does not rule out the possibility of a difficult intubation.

Features that have some value in predicting difficult intubation include:

Previous history of a difficult airway

- Look for a MedicAlert bracelet or similar. Ask about previous anaesthetic events and access patient medical records if available.

Body morphology

- Morbid obesity is an independent predictor of a difficult airway. The Fourth National Audit Project (NAP4) documented complications of airway management and showed that obesity was a factor in nearly half the airway management complications that led to harm.

Facial features

- Poor mouth opening – less than 4–5 cm or three finger breadths incisor to incisor (or gum to gum in edentulous patients) will reduce access and view of the larynx.
- Prominent upper incisors will restrict view and access. Jagged teeth may puncture the cuff of a tracheal tube.
- A high-arched palate reduces the space inside the mouth, compromising access during laryngoscopy.
- Receding mandible (see thyromental distance below).
- An inability to move the lower teeth in front of the upper teeth.
- Macroglossia reduces space within the mouth and makes the tongue harder to move.
- Facial trauma causing deranged facial anatomy. Bleeding into the soft tissues may distort the anatomy and normal colouration of the pharynx and larynx, making landmarks more difficult to identify. Fractures involving the temporomandibular joints may be particularly dangerous as they can prevent any mouth opening even after a neuromuscular blocker has been given. Paradoxically, unstable, and therefore mobile, facial bony injuries may facilitate laryngoscopy and subsequent intubation.

Neck

- Thyromental distance < 6–7 cm, or four finger breadths, from the top of the thyroid cartilage to the anterior border of the mandible with the neck in full extension implies a short mandible and/or a high larynx; both may impair the view at laryngoscopy or make intubation very difficult.
- Trauma – blunt trauma may rarely fracture the larynx, altering the anatomy and making it difficult to identify structures during laryngoscopy.
- Penetrating trauma may cause haematomas that displace the larynx, making the view and access difficult, yet are not visible externally.
- Infection causing either generalized swelling (e.g. pharyngitis, laryngitis, epiglottitis) or focal swelling (retropharyngeal abscess or quinsy) may cause obstruction.

- Tumours, previous surgery or radiotherapy may all alter normal anatomy and reduce soft tissue mobility.
- Reduced skeletal mobility will worsen the view of the larynx. The best views are obtained in adults with the head in extension and the neck in flexion. This is the 'sniffing the morning air' position, which aligns the airway axes and makes it easier to see the glottis (see Chapter 3). Reduced neck mobility may be present in presumed or actual cervical spine injury, the elderly, in patients with arthritis of the cervical spine, and in patients with previous neck injuries or surgery. During laryngoscopy with in-line stabilization of the neck and pressure applied to the cricoid cartilage the view of the glottis will be Cormack and Lehane grade 3 or 4 in 20% of cases. The use of videolaryngoscopy will reduce this incidence. In obese patients, women with large breasts or patients with severe fixed flexion neck deformities (e.g. ankylosing spondylitis), it may be difficult to get the laryngoscope blade into the mouth whilst mounted on the handle. In these cases the blade may have to be inserted separately or a specialist laryngoscope used (such as a polio blade or a fibre optic scope).

Mallampati and other scoring systems

A Mallampati score of I to IV is used to describe the view of the patient's tongue, faucial pillars, uvula and posterior pharynx (Figure 5.2). Scores of III or above are associated with limited views at laryngoscopy. To be valid, the assessment is undertaken with the patient seated in front of the practitioner with the head extended on a flexed neck. The patient is asked to open their mouth wide and protrude their tongue.

Other scoring systems (for example, the Simplified Predictive Intubation Difficulty Score (SPIDS), and the Simplified Airway Risk Index (SARI)) have been advocated. These use a combination of features in an attempt to improve the sensitivity and specificity of predicting a difficult airway, but they have had limited success. SARI uses a score derived from seven risk factors (mouth opening, thyromental distance, Mallampati score, neck mobility, ability to prognath, weight and history of difficult intubation) and is currently being evaluated in the elective anaesthesia population in an attempt to validate this form of assessment for predicting difficulty with intubation and BMV.

All these scoring systems require time, a compliant patient able to mobilize, and often prior knowledge of the patient. None of this may be available when dealing with an emergency airway, and they therefore have a limited role in pre-intubation airway assessment in this context.

Predicting a difficult cricothyroidotomy

Performing a surgical or needle cricothyroidotomy is a rescue procedure that may enable oxygenation of a patient in a 'can't intubate, can't oxygenate'

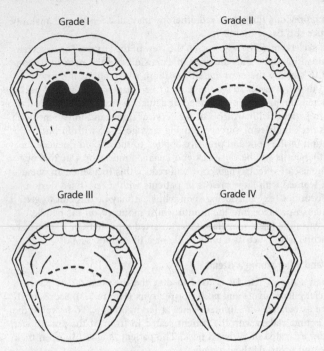

Figure 5.2 The Mallampati Score, modified by Samsoon and Young.

situation. These techniques rely on the cricothyroid membrane being accessible, which may not always be the case.

Features that may cause difficulty in accessing the cricothyroid membrane

- Obesity. A layer of subcutaneous tissues makes the anatomical landmarks ill-defined and difficult to locate.
- Neck immobility. Being unable to extend the head on the neck may restrict access, particularly in the obese or short-necked patient.
- Local trauma. Significant blunt or penetrating trauma may distort the anatomy, as may burns over the anterior neck.

HAVNO

A simple reminder for assessing predictors of a difficult airway is:

H History – including previous airway problems.

A Anatomy – features of the face, mouth, and teeth that may suggest intubation will be difficult.

V Visual clues – trauma, obesity, facial hair, age.

N Neck mobility and accessibility, including the presence of in-line stabilization.

O Opening of the mouth – less than three fingers suggests potential difficulty with intubation.

What to do if a difficult airway is predicted

Airway management in an emergency is more difficult than in elective practice, so the emergency airway practitioner must always be prepared for difficulty, even if not predicted. By using the approach described above, a difficult airway can often be anticipated so that, time allowing, rapid sequence induction is not undertaken in the absence of the most experienced available assistance unless the patient has life-threatening hypoxaemia or is deteriorating despite all possible basic airway interventions. The management of difficult and failed airway is described in Chapter 9.

Summary

- Always be prepared for a difficult airway.
- No single airway assessment tool is sufficiently sensitive or specific to reliably predict a difficult or easy airway.
- In some cases features of the patient's morphology and pathology enable a difficult airway to be predicted.
- Rarely, patients with no predictive features may be difficult or impossible to intubate using conventional techniques.
- Intubation is rarely so urgent that airway assessment is not possible; aim to undertake a pre-anaesthetic assessment in all but the most unusual cases, and document the findings.

Further reading

1 Cormack, R.S., Lehane, J. (1984) Difficult tracheal intubation in obstetrics. Anaesthesia; 39: 1105–11.

2 Bair, A.E., Filbin, M.R., Kulkarni, R.G., Walls, R.M. (2002) The failed intubation attempt in the emergency department: analysis of prevalence, rescue techniques, and personnel. J Emerg Med; 23: 131–40.

3 Graham, C.A., Beard, D., Oglesby, A.J. et al. (2003) Rapid sequence intubation in Scottish urban emergency departments. Emerg Med J; 20: 3–5.

4 Langeron, O., Masso, E., Huraux, C. et al. (2000) Prediction of difficult mask ventilation. Anesthesiology; 92: 1229–35.

5   Hasegawa, K., Shigemitsu, K., Hagiwara, Y. *et al.* (2012) Association between repeated intubation attempts and adverse events in emergency departments: an analysis of a multicenter prospective observational study. Ann Emerg Med; 60: 749–54.

6   Cook, T.M., Woodall, N., Harper, J. *et al.* (2011) Major complications of airway management in the UK: Results of the Fourth National Audit Project of the Royal College of Anaesthetists and the Difficult Airway Society. Part 2: intensive care and emergency departments. Br J Anaesth; 106: 632–42.

7   Walls, R.M., Brown, C.A., 3rd, Bair, A.E. *et al.* (2011) Emergency airway management: a multi-center report of 8937 emergency department intubations. J Emerg Med; 41: 347–54.

8   Kheterpal, S., Healy, D., Aziz, M.F. *et al.* (2013) Incidence, predictors, and outcome of difficult mask ventilation combined with difficult laryngoscopy. Anesthesiology; 119: 1360–9.

9   Sakles, J.C., Mosier, J., Chiu, S., Cosentino, M., Kalin, L. (2012) A comparison of the C-Mac videolaryngoscope to the Macintosh direct laryngoscope for intubation in the emergency department. Ann Emerg Med; 60: 739–48.

Chapter

6

Preparation for rapid sequence induction

Simon J. A. Chapman and Les Gordon

Objectives

The objectives of this chapter are to:

- Be able to prepare thoroughly for rapid sequence induction of anaesthesia (RSI) and tracheal intubation.
- Understand how to optimize pre-oxygenation and reduce the rate of desaturation after the onset of apnoea.
- Be able to position patients optimally to maximize the success of laryngoscopy and intubation.
- Understand how to assemble and check the equipment and drugs required for RSI and tracheal intubation.
- Be able to use appropriate monitoring and know its strengths and limitations.
- Understand the importance of reassessing the patient rapidly and ascertaining all the required information before undertaking RSI.
- Be familiar with use of pre-procedural checklists and team briefings, and understand their benefits.
- Be able to identify and use team resources appropriately to maximize team cooperation and understanding.

Introduction

Making the decision that a patient requires a rapid sequence induction (RSI) and tracheal intubation is the entry point to the sequence of preparation for this procedure. While there may be times when intubation of the patient needs to be achieved immediately, there are very few instances in which placement of the tracheal tube is so time critical that these basic preparatory steps cannot be followed. With a systematic approach and good team working these will take

Emergency Airway Management, Second Edition, ed. Andrew Burtenshaw, Jonathan Benger and Jerry Nolan. Published by Cambridge University Press. © College of Emergency Medicine, London, 2015.

only a few minutes, avoid many possible problems and complications, and increase the chance of success.

PEACH (Box 6.1) is a useful mnemonic.

Box 6.1 The PEACH mnemonic

Positioning
Equipment – including drugs
Attach – oxygen and monitoring
Checks – Pre-procedural checklist, resuscitation, brief history, intravenous
    access and neurology
Help – who is available and what are the abilities of the team?

Positioning

Optimal positioning of the patient for RSI and tracheal intubation is intended to:

- improve pre-oxygenation;
- decrease rate of desaturation following apnoea;
- improve grade of laryngeal view at laryngoscopy.

Approximately 25% of RSIs undertaken in the emergency department include stabilization of the spine, requiring the patient to be managed in a supine position. This is not ideal for achieving optimal pre-oxygenation or the best view at laryngoscopy. Therefore, in almost all other cases the patient is placed in an optimum intubating position, unless spinal deformity or arthritis makes this impractical or inadvisable.

Positioning for pre-oxygenation

When lying in the supine position it is difficult for a patient to take large breaths. Posterior lung tissue becomes prone to atelectasis, reducing the number of alveoli available for pre-oxygenation. This decreases the reservoir of oxygen contained within the lungs and therefore reduces the period an apnoeic patient is likely to maintain arterial blood oxygen saturation above 92%, which is known as the safe apnoea time. This effect is compounded in the obese (body mass index [BMI] > 30) and/or pregnant (> 20 weeks) patient. Managing patients in a head-up or reverse Trendelenburg position can significantly improve this situation. By displacing the weight of soft tissue from the anterior chest wall, the load on the thoracic cavity is decreased and the pressure of intra-abdominal contents on the diaphragm reduced. Both of these factors can increase the lung functional residual capacity and reduce atelectasis, thereby improving the effectiveness of pre-oxygenation.

Studies performed on patients pre-oxygenated in a 20° head-up position have demonstrated that it takes up to 90 seconds longer for arterial blood to desaturate from 100% to 95% when compared to controls pre-oxygenated in the supine position.

Obese patients receiving three minutes' pre-oxygenation in a 25° head-up position have shown blood oxygen partial pressures (P_aO_2) > 20% higher and take up to 50 seconds longer for arterial blood to desaturate from 100% to 92% when compared to pre-oxygenation in the supine position.

However, some hypotensive patients may not tolerate a head-up or reverse Trendelenburg position, and the effect on cerebral perfusion must be considered. In these cases, consider concurrent leg elevation (the scissor position) or fluid/inotropic support.

Positioning for intubation

Correct positioning of the patient's head and neck improves the view of the larynx at laryngoscopy and the likelihood of successful intubation. During laryngoscopy, alignment of the oral, pharyngeal and laryngeal axes in the 'sniffing the morning air' position can provide a clear view from the incisors to the laryngeal inlet (see Chapter 8).

Studies in obese patients have shown that achieving a position where the external auditory meatus is on the same horizontal plane as the sternal notch improves direct laryngoscopy. This is commonly referred to as the ramped position, and can be achieved with the trolley back elevated and a pillow under the occiput, by using proprietary ramp devices or by pillows alone. (See Figures 6.1 and 6.2)

The ramped position will facilitate both pre-oxygenation and intubation, and has been shown to be of benefit in obese and non-obese patients. Having achieved the appropriate ramped position for pre-oxygenation the patient does not require repositioning for intubation.

Equipment

Prepare and check thoroughly all equipment before undertaking any anaesthetic. These checks are the responsibility of the practitioner who will give the anaesthetic. This individual must be familiar with all the equipment and check it adequately. Many of these checks may be undertaken in advance as part of a routine daily check. A systematic approach is recommended (Box 6.2); equipment is placed in a logical sequence and positioned conveniently within easy reach. Equipment for managing a failed intubation must also be readily available and checked.

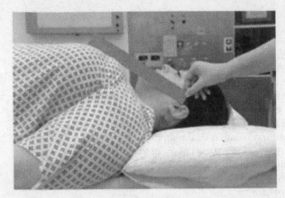

Figure 6.1 Supine patient without ramping (Photograph courtesy of Alma Medical).

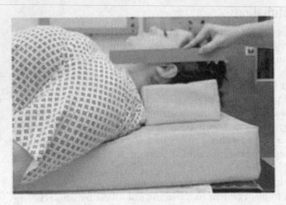

Figure 6.2 Proprietary devices or pillows may be used to align the thorax, shoulders, head and neck to improve the view at laryngoscopy (Photograph courtesy of Alma Medical).

As discussed in the Fourth National Audit Project (NAP4) report, there are advantages to having a standardized airway management trolley in all critical care areas of the hospital. This will promote familiarity with equipment and improve the ease with which other practitioners can assist in airway management.

Trolley

Check the patient trolley/stretcher to ensure operation of the height adjustment and mechanism for rapid tilting. Position it optimally to ensure access to the patient for intubation, effortless view of monitoring and immediate availability of the anaesthetic equipment.

Suction

When obstructed, suction should generate a negative pressure of 400 cmH$_2$O within ten seconds. Ensure it is immediately accessible during management of the airway; it is usually placed under the pillow on the right side to facilitate use whilst the laryngoscope is positioned with the left hand.

Rigid catheters are required for suctioning of the upper airway (e.g. Yankauer type), and flexible suction catheters for suctioning down the tracheal tube after placement.

Oxygen delivery apparatus

Check oxygen delivery systems for patency and ability to generate positive pressure for ventilation, including the high-pressure injector (see Box 6.2). Check also the function of adjustable pressure limiting (APL) valves.

Connect a heat and moisture exchanger (HME) filter to the breathing system; it prevents contamination of ventilation equipment and helps to warm and humidify the oxygen-enriched air in the trachea during ventilation. Use a twist and push movement to check that all connections are hand tight.

Backup oxygen supply

Ensure that a separate oxygen cylinder is available, that it is functioning and is at least three-quarters full.

Airway adjuncts

Airway adjuncts, including several sizes of oral and nasopharyngeal airways, should be available. Take care when removing these devices from wrappers; avoid sealing the ends of the airways with a thin film of polythene, and ensure that no unrelated equipment (e.g. cannula caps) is able to inadvertently enter the airway devices.

Laryngoscopes
Direct laryngoscopy

The curved Macintosh laryngoscope blade is commonly available in sizes 3 (short) and 4 (long); use the size 4 blade in all but the smallest adult patients. Check that the laryngoscope light is adequately bright before starting an RSI. Alternative laryngoscope blades such as the McCoy blade (which enables further elevation of the epiglottis using the lever on the tip of the curved blade) or the Miller straight-bladed laryngoscope are useful alternatives. Use of these alternative blades requires adequate training; they should never be used for the first time in a difficult situation.

Box 6.2 Equipment for rapid sequence induction and tracheal intubation

Basic resuscitation equipment:
- tilting trolley/stretcher;
- oxygen delivery apparatus, including mask with reservoir and oxygen tubing;
- nasal cannulae for apnoeic oxygenation;
- suction:
  - wide-bore suction tubing;
  - rigid suction catheter;
  - flexible suction catheter – sized appropriately for airway equipment;
- airway adjuncts:
  - nasopharyngeal airway (sizes 6 mm and 7 mm);
  - oropharyngeal airway (sizes 2, 3 and 4);
- intravenous access equipment;
- monitoring:
  - pulse oximetry;
  - waveform capnometer;
  - three-lead ECG;
  - non-invasive blood pressure (NIBP).

Advanced airway equipment:
- pre-oxygenation/ventilation breathing system:
  - Mapleson C or equivalent anaesthetic breathing system;
  - bag-mask apparatus with reservoir bag and oxygen tubing;
  - filter (heat and moisture exchanger);
- drugs – in labelled syringes;
- laryngoscope handles and blades (sizes 3 and 4 for adults);
- videolaryngoscope of choice (if available);
- Magill's forceps;
- intubating stylet, bougie and lubricating gel;
- tracheal tubes in a range of sizes;
- 20 mL syringe;
- tie and adhesive tape;
- equipment for patient ventilation:
  - catheter mount;
  - waveform capnometer;
  - ventilator.

Failed intubation equipment:
- supraglottic airway device of choice in appropriate range of sizes:
  - +/– 50 mL syringe to inflate device if required;
  - lubricating gel;
- surgical cricothyroidotomy set;
- needle cricothyroidotomy kit with high-pressure injector.

Indirect laryngoscopy

There is now a wide variety of devices, such as videolaryngoscopes, that enable indirect laryngoscopy. Such devices can improve the grade of laryngoscopic view and reduce intubation difficulty, particularly in patients with an immobilized cervical spine or other cause of a difficult airway. However, there are some limitations of indirect laryngoscopy; intubation can take longer using one of these devices than with direct laryngoscopy; an indirect view can be obscured by blood or other fluids in the airway and they should be used only by practitioners who are fully trained and competent in their use.

Tracheal tubes

The tracheal tube sizes recommended for adults are 7.0 or 7.5 mm for women and 8.0 mm for men; however, a range of tracheal tube sizes should be available. Use a smaller than normal diameter tube if mucosal oedema is expected, e.g. following inhalational burns. While tubes are normally cut to length (22–24 cm for women, 24–26 cm for men), if facial swelling is likely, e.g. with burns, blunt facial trauma or anaphylaxis, leave the tube uncut. Ensure a syringe is available to fill the cuff with air and check this before RSI to ensure that it does not leak.

Bougies and stylets

The bougie and stylet are very useful aids to intubation. If the view at laryngoscopy is less than perfect (grade 3 or a difficult grade 2) it may be difficult or impossible to pass a tracheal tube directly through the vocal cords. Instead, an intubating bougie can be inserted behind the epiglottis and into the trachea, enabling a tracheal tube to be railroaded into position over the bougie. Some practitioners prefer to use an intubating stylet; the rigidity of this device enables the tube to be shaped to bring the tip more anterior, forming a J shape, which facilitates intubation. For further information see Chapter 8.

Ventilation system

Carefully check the ventilation system and all of its connections according to the manufacturer's instructions. Check the system functions normally and check the settings of the high (e.g. potential obstruction) and low (e.g. potential disconnection) pressure alarms, the ventilation mode, respiratory rate, tidal volume, inspiratory:expiratory (I:E) ratio and positive end expiratory pressure (PEEP) (see Chapter 10 for further information).

Equipment for failed intubation

Check the equipment for failed intubation and place it in an easily accessible location during all intubations. Ideally, this equipment will be available on a standardized difficult airway trolley.

Drugs

The choice of drugs for induction of anaesthesia and maintenance of sedation and analgesia are described in detail in Chapter 7. Once the drugs are selected, prepare them in appropriately sized, clearly labelled syringes. Include the drugs that may be required for treatment of any hypotension associated with the RSI.

Attach

Oxygen

To achieve optimal pre-oxygenation give high-flow oxygen to the patient in all but the most unusual circumstances; use a breathing system that will maximize oxygen delivery. The minimum requirement is high-flow oxygen (15 L min^{-1}) through a well-fitting mask with a functioning oxygen reservoir. Although turning the flow meter beyond 15 L min^{-1} may further increase the inspired concentration of oxygen, the flow delivered will be unknown and equipment safety may be compromised. Pre-oxygenation can be achieved using a self-inflating bag-mask. The practitioner also has to maintain a good mask seal during the stressful moments of preparing for RSI. If the seal is inadequate, room air will be entrained, decreasing the inspired oxygen concentration. An effective alternative is an anaesthetic breathing system, such as a Mapleson C circuit. These can deliver high oxygen concentrations, require minimal inspiratory effort and the oxygen reservoir bag provides a clear view of respiratory effort. However, a higher level of skill is required to use these devices safely and effectively. In patients with significant lung disease causing hypoxaemia, pre-oxygenation may be achieved optimally using non-invasive respiratory support (CPAP or NIPPV), particularly if the patient requires this treatment to maintain oxygenation prior to RSI.

Pre-oxygenation is normally undertaken while the patient is breathing spontaneously. When drugs are injected the patient is rendered apnoeic and their haemoglobin will begin to desaturate. Apnoeic oxygenation provides continuous oxygen delivery during this period and throughout the intubation process. Well-fitting nasal cannulae providing high-flow oxygen can slow the desaturation process by improving the oxygen concentration in the proximal divisions of the respiratory tract. This may decrease the risk of hypoxaemia, provided that there is no upper airway obstruction. The nasal cannulae are fitted to the patient during pre-oxygenation and the flow increased from 4 L min^{-1} to 15 L min^{-1} as intubation drugs are administered. The cannulae remain *in situ* until successful intubation is achieved.

Monitoring

The Association of Anaesthetists of Great Britain and Ireland has defined minimum recommended standards of monitoring, which are required wherever anaesthesia is administered (see Further reading section). These standards apply as much outside the operating room as they do within it, and include the monitoring of:

- inspired oxygen concentration (F_iO_2);
- capnography;
- pulse oximetry;
- non-invasive blood pressure;
- continuous electrocardiograph (ECG).

Anyone carrying out anaesthesia should understand the rationale behind these recommendations and the major strengths and limitations of the different monitors that they are likely to use on a regular basis.

Oxygen analyzer

Use an oxygen analyzer to ensure adequate delivery of oxygen whenever positive pressure ventilation is undertaken. Measurement of F_iO_2 is often achieved in combination with measurement of end tidal CO_2.

Electrocardiograph

ECG monitoring is an easy and non-invasive method for detecting changes in heart rate and rhythm. Changes in morphology of the ECG may indicate myocardial ischaemia or electrolyte disturbances such as hypokalaemia or hyperkalaemia. The ECG gives no indication of cardiac output.

Non-invasive blood pressure

Measurement of the blood pressure alone provides limited information about tissue perfusion. However, trends may indicate physiological change and sudden hypotension may warn of an acute life-threatening event such as anaphylaxis or tension pneumothorax. An inflatable cuff of the correct size on the upper arm measures non-invasive blood pressure. Measure the blood pressure more frequently when physiological change is anticipated, such as at the induction of anaesthesia. These machines are notoriously unreliable at the extremes of pressure and with irregular rhythms. In these circumstances, direct measurement of blood pressure using an intra-arterial cannula is preferable.

Pulse oximetry

The nature of the plethysmograph trace gives information about the state of the peripheral circulation. Pulsatile flow is required for correct function; in low flow states the information displayed by the pulse oximeter may be inaccurate. While the pulse oximeter indicates haemoglobin oxygen saturation, it may not reflect adequacy of ventilation of the patient; information should be interpreted in conjunction with capnography and arterial blood gas analysis.

Capnography

The Fourth National Audit Project (NAP4) provides further support to the absolute necessity of having quantitative waveform capnography in use whenever a patient is intubated. The presence of expired CO_2 is the most reliable way of confirming placement of a tracheal tube in a major airway (examination and auscultation are required to ensure it is not in a bronchus). If CO_2 is not detected, assume oesophageal intubation and immediately remove the tube.

Some systems require warming up before use, and this must be undertaken before any intubation attempt. Although trends in CO_2 may indicate the adequacy of ventilation, the absolute value may correlate poorly with the partial pressure of CO_2 measured from an arterial blood sample. The results of blood gas analysis take precedence in assessing ventilatory adequacy. A sudden decrease in CO_2 may indicate displacement of the tracheal tube or a reduced cardiac output. Even in cardiac arrest and very low flow states, the capnograph trace retains a distinctive, if attenuated, square waveform, particularly when effective cardiopulmonary resuscitation is ongoing. Therefore, an entirely flat quantitative capnograph trace indicates failed intubation or a dislodged tracheal tube, rather than cardiac arrest.

Checks

Checklists and team briefings

Emergency RSI and tracheal intubation represents a complex sequence of steps carried out by a team of individuals with the aim of achieving definitive airway control. This process should be coordinated by a team leader with the aim of avoiding any complications or untoward events.

Teams may comprise individuals from the same department who often work together, or may include staff from different disciplines who do not.

Pre-procedural checklists and team briefings reduce errors and untoward incidents. Use an intubation checklist for all intubations of critically ill patients and identify backup plans.

An example is provided in Appendix 3.

Resuscitation

During resuscitation, review airway, breathing and circulation (ABC), paying particular attention to any potentially reversible problems. Request any relevant laboratory tests and optimize the drug treatment of any medical conditions, including analgesia, if appropriate. Document all baseline physiology.

Box 6.3 AMPLE history

- **A**llergies
- **M**edications
- **P**MHx (past medical history)
- **L**ast:
  - anaesthetic (complications?);
  - meal;
  - tetanus;
- **E**vents:
  - Leading up to this situation.

Brief history

Review a brief history (such as the AMPLE history described in Box 6.3) to obtain information relevant to clinical decisions. Although it is usual to enquire about the last meal, in practice, all emergency cases are considered to have a full stomach.

Intravenous access

Ensure that there are two functioning intravenous (IV) lines before giving any anaesthetic drugs. Failure of the sole IV line during an RSI is dangerous.

Neurology

Undertake a brief neurological examination before induction of anaesthesia (and therefore abolition of neurological signs). This will include assessment of GCS, pupil signs and motor response for each limb. Look for diaphragmatic breathing, inappropriate vasodilatation or priapism. Document all neurological findings.

Help

Call for help

An appropriately experienced individual should be present before undertaking advanced airway management in a critically ill patient. If RSI is anticipated, summon expert help immediately. The presence of a senior emergency airway practitioner from the earliest opportunity is ideal.

Organize team members

Rapid sequence induction of anaesthesia outside the operating room requires a minimum of three or four staff. One practitioner takes responsibility for the airway and another oversees the clinical care of the patient. It is essential that the airway practitioner is accompanied by an assistant who is capable of applying cricoid pressure correctly, and who has knowledge of the equipment and techniques to be used, including the plan for difficult or failed intubation. A fourth member of staff will be required to undertake manual in-line stabilization of the cervical spine, if this is indicated.

Good team leadership is vitally important (see Chapter 13). The key skills of good leadership include:

- briefing of new team members;
- delegation;
- allocation and agreement of roles;
- task distribution (and support if required);
- coordination and communication.

Review and feedback

A debrief of team performance after the event provides an opportunity for reflection and learning.

Summary

Thorough preparation before undertaking RSI and tracheal intubation will minimize unexpected problems and facilitate a smooth and successful procedure.

Acknowledgement

This chapter has been updated from the first edition chapter, which was written by Nicki Maran, Neil Nichol and Simon Leigh-Smith.

Further reading

1   Association of Anaesthetists of Great Britain and Ireland (2007) *Recommendations for Standards of Monitoring*, 4th edn. London: Association of Anaesthetists of Great Britain and Ireland. Available at: http://www.aagbi.org/sites/default/files/ standardsofmonitoring07.pdf (accessed November 2014).

2   NAP4. Fourth National Audit Project of The Royal College of Anaesthetists and The Difficult Airway Society. (2011) *Major Complications of Airway Management in the United Kingdom.* ISBN 978-1-900936-03-3.

3   Weingart, S.D., Levitan, R.M. (2012) Preoxygenation and prevention of desaturation during emergency airway management. Ann Emerg Med; 59: 165–75.

Chapter 7

Pharmacology of emergency airway drugs

Shirley Lindsay and Jonathan Benger

Objectives

The objectives of this chapter are to:

- Be familiar with the choice of induction, analgesic and neuromuscular blocking drugs.
- Understand the advantages and disadvantages of drugs used in emergency airway management.
- Understand the basic pharmacology of these drugs.
- Be aware of the possible complications caused by these drugs.

Introduction

The term 'triad of anaesthesia' is used to describe the components of a balanced anaesthetic:

- hypnosis;
- analgesia;
- muscle relaxation.

The pharmacology of drugs used commonly in emergency airway management will be considered under these three headings.

In unmodified rapid sequence induction an analgesic is omitted and the patient is given a pre-calculated dose of induction drug and neuromuscular blocker only. The rationale behind this is that, should intubation fail, the patient will recover from anaesthesia and paralysis quickly, returning to spontaneous ventilation. Opioids, particularly in high doses, may prolong the time to spontaneous ventilation. Some patients may have received analgesia before the induction of anaesthesia (e.g. for pain relief in trauma), and

Emergency Airway Management, Second Edition, ed. Andrew Burtenshaw, Jonathan Benger and Jerry Nolan. Published by Cambridge University Press. © College of Emergency Medicine, London, 2015.

under some circumstances it is appropriate to consider modifying an RSI to include a carefully selected dose of opioid given before the induction drug (e.g. RSI in the presence of raised intracranial pressure: see Chapter 11.2). Opioids are also useful after intubation, when they may be used in combination with a hypnotic to maintain anaesthesia and reduce sympathetic stimulation.

Midazolam is not considered an induction drug in the UK. Hypotension, bradycardia and long duration of action limit its usefulness as an induction drug in emergency airway management. However, midazolam may occasionally be given by an experienced practitioner to sedate an agitated and uncooperative patient to facilitate the process of RSI. It is also used for procedural sedation, and is therefore included in the hypnosis section.

Any modification of a standard rapid sequence induction will alter the pharmacodynamic response to induction drugs. Therefore the risks and benefits of RSI modification should be considered for individual patients.

Hypnosis
Induction drugs

The ideal anaesthetic induction drug would induce anaesthesia smoothly and rapidly without causing pain on injection. It would cause minimal depression of the respiratory and cardiovascular systems, and protect the cerebral circulation. Recovery would be rapid and the drug would have no adverse effects. Unfortunately, such a drug does not exist, and the attributes and limitations of available drugs, as well as the condition of the patient, will determine the final choice. Familiarity with the properties of a specific drug is also very important. It is not appropriate to use an unfamiliar drug for the first time in an emergency.

All induction drugs have the potential to cause hypotension to a greater or lesser extent, particularly when the patient is physiologically compromised.

In the UK, one of four induction drugs is used in emergency RSI: these are summarized in Table 7.1, and described in more detail subsequently. However, this manual does not attempt to provide a comprehensive account of the properties of individual drugs and readers are referred to pharmacological texts for further information.

Etomidate has fewer adverse effects on the cardiovascular system than thiopental or propofol and, particularly in the presence of hypovolaemia, will cause less hypotension than these drugs. In critically ill patients a single dose of etomidate causes adrenal suppression for up to 24 hours: the clinical significance of this is unclear, but it may be a cause of subsequent morbidity and mortality. Do not use etomidate in septic patients. Many practitioners prefer to use ketamine, thiopental or propofol, even in hypovolaemic patients, but this necessitates considerable experience of these drugs, and a carefully considered dose reduction, particularly if propofol is used. Where

Table 7.1 Summary of the four commonly used induction drugs

Induction drug	Dose	Onset of anaesthesia	Recovery	Cardiovascular depression	Specific effects
Thiopental	2–7 mg kg^{-1}	5–15 seconds	5–15 minutes	++	• Cerebroprotective action • Useful in isolated head injury • Effective anticonvulsant • Histamine release
Etomidate	0.3 mg kg^{-1}	5–15 seconds	5–15 minutes	+	• Relatively little cardiovascular depression • Myoclonic movements on induction • Adrenal suppression
Propofol	1.5–2.5 mg kg^{-1}	20–40 seconds	5–10 minutes	+++	• Marked hypotension in cardiovascular compromise • Induction drug most commonly used in elective anaesthesia • Pain on injection • Involuntary movements on induction • Anticonvulsant properties
Ketamine	1–2 mg kg^{-1}	15–30 seconds	15–30 minutes	Minimal	• Dissociative state • Potent analgesic • Hypertension • Emergence phenomena e.g. agitation, hallucinations • Bronchodilator • Useful in acute asthma, hypovolaemic trauma and burns

time allows, the placement of an arterial cannula is invaluable during RSI to provide accurate and continuous blood pressure measurement.

Ketamine is a useful induction drug in some circumstances: it is a bronchodilator, causes less hypotension and respiratory depression than the other induction drugs, and is a potent analgesic. The use of ketamine for induction is increasing, especially in critically ill patients, particularly trauma patients, and earlier concerns about adverse effects in patients with traumatic brain injury have not been demonstrated in practice. It can, however, cause hypertension. At the time of induction, the clinician must determine the clinical priorities for each patient, bearing in mind the benefits, but also the potential pitfalls, of each induction drug.

Etomidate

Indications

- Induction of anaesthesia in the haemodynamically compromised patient.

Induction characteristics

- 5–15 seconds onset;
- 5–15 minutes full recovery;
- myoclonic movement on injection (may be mistaken for seizures);
- pain on injection.

Physiological effects

- hypnotic;
- relative haemodynamic stability;
- attenuation of the increase in ICP that accompanies laryngoscopy;
- reduced cerebral blood flow;
- reduced cerebral oxygen demand;
- adrenocortical suppression; must never be given by infusion;
- do not use in a patient with sepsis.

Dose

- 0.3 mg kg^{-1} IV.

Propofol

Indications

- most commonly used induction drug in elective anaesthesia;
- can be used by infusion for maintenance of anaesthesia or sedation;
- sedation in intubated patients on ICU or during transport.

Induction characteristics

- slow onset (20–40 seconds) can lead to overdose;
- rapid return of consciousness.

Physiological effects

- hypotension is common, and may be severe in cardiovascular compromise and the elderly; it is caused mainly by vasodilatation, but also by a direct myocardial depressant effect;
- apnoea after induction dose;
- pain on injection with some preparations (reduced if 2 mL of 1% lidocaine is mixed with the induction dose or injected before induction);
- occasional severe bradycardia;
- induction often associated with involuntary movements, but anticonvulsant properties have been demonstrated on EEG studies.

Dose

- 1.5–2.5 mg kg^{-1} IV.

Thiopental sodium

Indications

- haemodynamically stable patient with:
  - isolated head injury;
  - seizures.

Induction characteristics

- 5–15 seconds onset;
- 5–15 minutes to recovery.

Physiological effects

- neuro-inhibition (at barbiturate receptor as part of GABA–receptor complex);
- cerebroprotective, because of a dose-dependant decrease in:
  - cerebral metabolic oxygen consumption;
  - cerebral blood flow;
  - ICP;
- maintenance of cerebral perfusion pressure;
- venodilation;
- myocardial depression;
- central respiratory depression;
- causes histamine release; can induce or exacerbate bronchospasm.

Dose

- 2–7 mg kg^{-1} IV;
- dose reduced to 1.5–2 mg kg^{-1} IV in haemodynamically unstable patients and the elderly.

Ketamine

Indications

- trauma, particularly burns;
- septic shock;
- cardiovascularly compromised patient;
- severe bronchospasm.

Induction characteristics

- 15–30 seconds onset when given IV;
- lack of a defined end-point makes dose calculation difficult;
- excitatory phenomena.

Physiological effects

- profound analgesia;
- sedation;
- dissociative state;
- amnesia (less than benzodiazepines);
- central sympathetic stimulation leading to:
  - . increased heart rate;
  - . increased blood pressure;
- bronchial smooth muscle relaxation;
- myocardial depression (in doses >1.5 mg kg^{-1});
- respiratory depression – dose related;
- enhanced laryngeal reflexes, with potential for laryngospasm;
- secretions increased – pharyngeal and bronchial;
- emergence phenomena:
  - . commoner in adults;
  - . reduced by pre-treatment with midazolam.

Dose

- 1–2 mg kg^{-1} IV;
- 5 mg kg^{-1} IM.

Midazolam

Midazolam is a water-soluble benzodiazepine that has anxiolytic, sedative and anticonvulsant properties. At physiological pH midazolam is lipid-soluble and reaches the central nervous system quickly. It has a shorter duration of action than most other benzodiazepines but causes profound, and sometimes prolonged, anterograde amnesia.

Indications

- procedural sedation;
- sedation of an agitated or uncooperative patient prior to RSI;
- ongoing patient sedation post-intubation (often with an opioid);
- reduction of side effects associated with ketamine.

Induction characteristics

- onset over 2 minutes;
- plasma half life is 2–6 hours, but the effects may be prolonged in elderly or debilitated patients;
- substantial variations in bioavailability have been reported.

Physiological effects

- sedation;
- anterograde amnesia;
- respiratory depression;
- minimal cardiovascular depression in lower sedative doses (but may cause bradycardia as well as hypotension in higher doses);
- vertigo and dizziness;
- visual disturbances and nausea;
- confusion in the elderly.

Dose

- $0.02–0.08$ mg kg^{-1} IV usually achieves effective patient sedation.

The elderly

The elderly require special consideration. Those over 65 years form a significant proportion of patients requiring emergency RSI and tracheal intubation. They are more likely than younger patients to have comorbidities, and safe RSI, sedation or anaesthesia requires knowledge of the pharmacokinetics and pharmacodynamics in the elderly.

The normal ageing process is associated with a degeneration of structure and function of organs and tissues, but the rate at which this occurs is variable, and depends more on biological than chronological age. The elderly are more likely to be dehydrated, which increases the hypotensive effects of anaesthetic induction drugs.

A reduced stroke volume and cardiac output prolongs the arm–brain circulation time for a drug and can increase the likelihood of overdose if induction is not modified. Cardiac reserve is diminished and hypotension more likely.

Consider carefully the drug dose and speed of administration. CNS changes include a reduction in neurotransmitter synthesis and a less effective blood–brain barrier. Reductions in plasma albumin concentration with reduced drug binding contribute to the elderly patient being more sensitive to the effects of anaesthetic drugs and opioids. Impaired renal function and dehydration raise the likelihood of hyperkalaemia at presentation, and will reduce the clearance of some drugs.

Analgesia

Opioids

Although not recommended as part of the classic rapid sequence induction technique, use of opioids will attenuate the cardiovascular responses to laryngoscopy and intubation. This may be particularly valuable if intracranial pressure is raised (see Chapter 11.2), where the patient is very hypertensive or has ischaemic heart disease. Where opioids are used, the required dose of induction drug will be reduced.

Many opioids have a relatively slow onset of action. The respiratory depression caused by opioids may be troublesome if intubation fails, because the patient may remain apnoeic despite recovery from neuromuscular blockade; if necessary, reversal of the opioid with naloxone will restore spontaneous breathing.

Fentanyl is a potent synthetic opioid which has a relatively fast onset (2–5 min) and short duration of action (30–60 min after a single dose). Its effects on the cardiovascular system are minimal, although large doses will cause bradycardia. Fentanyl (usual dose 2–3 mcg kg^{-1} IV) will reduce the hypertensive response, and offset the increase in intracranial pressure caused by laryngoscopy and intubation, providing that two to three minutes have elapsed between giving the drug and intubation.

Alfentanil (usual dose 10–20 mcg kg^{-1} IV) produces the same effects as fentanyl, but its peak action occurs after just 90 seconds and duration is 5–10 minutes: these characteristics make it ideal for attenuating the response to laryngoscopy and intubation.

If fentanyl or alfentanil are given, reduce the dose of induction drug (Table 7.2).

Neuromuscular blocking drugs

Suxamethonium

Suxamethonium (1.5–2 mg kg^{-1}) produces a dense neuromuscular block of rapid onset and short duration. It remains the drug of choice for neuromuscular blockade during RSI, although use of high-dose rocuronium is increasing for this purpose. Initial depolarization at the neuromuscular junction causes muscle fasciculation within 15 seconds (although this is not

Table 7.2 Commonly used opioids

	Alfentanil	Fentanyl	Morphine
Onset (minutes)	1	3	5
Duration (minutes)	10	40	180
Bolus dose	10–20 mcg kg^{-1}	2–3 mcg kg^{-1}	100 mcg kg^{-1}
Physiological effects	Analgesia. Respiratory depression. Anaesthesia at higher doses	Analgesia. Respiratory depression. Anaesthesia at higher doses	Analgesia. Respiratory depression.
Main side effects	Muscle rigidity. Bradycardia. Hypotension	Muscle rigidity. Bradycardia	Hypotension
Metabolism and excretion	Rapid liver metabolism	Liver metabolism	Renal clearance of active liver metabolites
Histamine release	No histamine release	Minimal histamine release	Significant histamine release

always seen) and complete paralysis follows after 45–60 seconds. Spontaneous return of muscle activity follows after metabolism of the drug by pseudocholinesterase.

Suxamethonium has significant side effects (see below).

Use

- remains the first line drug for muscular paralysis during rapid sequence induction.

Effects

- 10–15 seconds fasciculation;
- 45–60 seconds paralysis;
- 3–5 minutes first return of respiratory activity;
- 5–10 minutes return of effective spontaneous ventilation.

Contra-indications

- ECG changes suggesting hyperkalaemia;
- significant risk of hyperkalaemia (see Table 7.3).

Side effects

- hyperkalaemia;
- bradycardia;
- muscle fasciculation;
- muscle pain;
- histamine release;
- anaphylaxis;
- trigger drug for malignant hyperpyrexia in susceptible individuals;
- trismus/masseter spasm;
- prolonged neuromuscular blockade.

Dose

- 1.5–2 mg kg^{-1} IV.

Hyperkalaemia

After injecting suxamethonium, the plasma potassium concentration is increased by up to 0.5 mmol L^{-1}, even in normal subjects. If the plasma potassium concentration is 6.0 mmol L^{-1} or higher the increase may precipitate arrhythmias, or even cardiac arrest. The increase in potassium concentration may be greatly exaggerated in patients with certain pathological conditions, particularly demyelinating conditions, desquamating skin conditions, major trauma, burns and several other pathologies where loss of muscle excitation secondary to denervation, immobilization or inflammation leads to up-regulation of immature acetylcholine (Ach) receptors throughout the whole muscle membrane. Depolarization of these Ach receptors by suxamethonium can cause life-threatening hyperkalaemia. Although there are recognized periods of maximum risk for patients with these conditions (Table 7.3), the exact duration of the risk period is unpredictable and an alternative to suxamethonium should be considered in each case.

Bradycardia

Suxamethonium may cause bradycardia, particularly if large or repeated doses are given: children are most at risk. This should be anticipated, and atropine must be available. Children do not need to be pre-treated with atropine routinely, but draw up the correct dose (0.02 mg kg^{-1}) and be ready to give it whenever a child is anaesthetized.

Table 7.3 Pre-existing conditions in which suxamethonium may cause significant hyperkalaemia, and the periods of highest risk

Condition	Period of highest risk
Burns	2 days to 6 months
Peripheral neuropathy	5 days to 6 months
Spinal cord injury	5 days to 6 months, but may represent permanently increased risk
Upper motor neurone lesions or structural brain damage, including multiple sclerosis and stroke	5 days to 6 months, but may represent permanently increased risk
Muscular dystrophy/myopathies	Continuing
Severe trauma, infection and certain skin conditions	Dependent on severity and duration

Muscle fasciculation

The muscle fasciculation caused by suxamethonium can increase intracranial, intraocular and intragastric pressure. This effect is not significant when an adequate dose of an induction drug is given concurrently.

Muscle pain

This is most likely to occur 12–24 hours after giving suxamethonium to fit young patients and those who mobilize quickly after anaesthesia. It is seldom a clinical problem in patients undergoing emergency anaesthesia.

Histamine release

This will occur to a greater or lesser extent in all patients, and can cause significant hypotension.

Prolonged neuromuscular block

With repeated doses of suxamethonium the characteristics of the neuromuscular block change, and paralysis may be prolonged. In practice this should not be a problem as repeated doses of suxamethonium are rarely indicated. The action of suxamethonium may also be prolonged in the presence of organophosphate poisoning or cocaine use, when neuromuscular blockade may last 20–30 minutes. In patients with low or abnormal pseudocholinesterase activity, muscle paralysis after a dose of suxamethonium may last for several hours ('sux' apnoea). Treatment for this condition involves continued ventilation (including sedation) until normal neuromuscular activity returns.

Non-depolarizing muscle relaxants

In situations when suxamethonium is contra-indicated, rocuronium 1.0–1.2 mg kg^{-1} can be used for modified rapid sequence induction, and will enable intubation after 60 seconds. This dose will cause paralysis for about an hour. Anaphylaxis to rocuronium occurs, but is less common than anaphylaxis to suxamethonium. Some experienced practitioners favour a modified RSI using rocuronium instead of suxamethonium, and this has been further encouraged by the introduction of sugammadex (see below). However, it should not be assumed that sugammadex will automatically rescue a practitioner from a 'can't intubate, can't oxygenate' situation, and high-dose rocuronium is therefore most suited to a patient where the option to wake up is considered non-viable, even if intubation cannot be achieved, and where difficult intubation is considered unlikely. For this reason, RSI using rocuronium is best undertaken by senior staff, and with an acceptance that timely progression to surgical airway may be required (Table 7.4).

Sugammadex

If rocuronium has been chosen as the primary neuromuscular blocker for RSI its effect can be reversed rapidly with sugammadex given 3 minutes after rocuronium. This has potential benefits, but should be approached with caution.

Sugammadex is a cyclodextrin that encapsulates and then inactivates aminosteroid neuromuscular blocking drugs, including rocuronium. It forms a complex with the muscle relaxant in the plasma, thus reducing its ability to bind with receptors at the neuromuscular junction. Because one molecule of neuromuscular blocking drug binds to one molecule of sugammadex, the dose of sugammadex required depends on the extent of neuromuscular blockade to be reversed. For example, immediate reversal of rocuronium after RSI requires a large dose of sugammadex (i.e. 16 mg kg^{-1}). In the obese patient, the dose should be based on actual body weight.

Most patients will have a recovery of neuromuscular function by 3 minutes. However this potential benefit should be balanced against the following considerations:

- Patient oxygenation is an absolute priority.
- Sugammadex is costly, and therefore it is rarely drawn up until it is known that it will definitely be required. Studies have shown it can take up to 7 minutes from a decision to give sugammadex to actual injection; this is in addition to the time spent on several intubation attempts.
- Side effects include hypersensitivity, effects on haemostasis (with an increased risk of bleeding in some patient groups) and bradycardia.

Table 7.4 Commonly used non-depolarizing neuromuscular blockers

	Atracurium besylate	Vecuronium bromide	Rocuronium bromide
Onset (minutes)	3–5	3–5	1
Duration (minutes)	20–35	20–35	30–40
Loading dose	0.3 to 0.5 mg kg^{-1}	0.05 to 0.1 mg kg^{-1}	0.6 to 1.0 mg kg^{-1}
Infusion rate	5 to 10 mcg kg^{-1} min^{-1}	1 to 2 mcg kg^{-1} min^{-1}	2 to 8 mcg kg^{-1} min^{-1}
Metabolism/ excretion	Hofmann elimination	Hepatic/biliary	Hepatic/renal
Notes	Histamine release, less accumulation	Cardio-stable	Rapid onset

- The use of sugammadex for immediate reversal of rocuronium in children and adolescents has not been investigated, and so is not recommended.

Other non-depolarizing neuromuscular blockers are unlikely to be used during RSI, but may be used for maintaining muscle relaxation following recovery from suxamethonium.

Potential drug-related complications

The following complications can occur for the first time during emergency anaesthesia, but in some cases may be anticipated from the history of previous anaesthetics, allergies or family reactions to anaesthetic. This emphasizes the importance – even in emergencies – of thorough preparation, including a brief history where possible. Other information may also be found amongst the patient's possessions, wallet or MedicAlert jewellery.

Malignant hyperthermia

Malignant hyperthermia (MH) is a life-threatening disorder of skeletal muscle calcium homeostasis. Its inheritance is autosomal dominant, with an incidence of around 1 in 30,000. The most common triggers are suxamethonium and volatile anaesthetics. Diagnosis can be difficult, and it may present insidiously over hours or as an acute life-threatening event at induction. Hyperthermia itself may be a late feature, as are the effects of rhabdomyolysis. Signs can be considered in two groups: direct muscle effects and the effects of increased metabolism. Masseter muscle spasm (MMS) may indicate MH, and can be the only sign of it, but is not pathognomonic since it also occurs in a few normal patients, especially children, after suxamethonium. After injection of suxamethonium, MMS will cause trismus at a time when relaxation would normally have been expected, but it does not usually persist long enough to hinder attempts at intubation. Treat prolonged MMS as a potential case of MH.

The most common signs of increased metabolism are:

- unexplained increasing E_TCO_2;
- concomitant tachycardia and arrhythmias;
- decreasing oxygen saturation;
- flushing.

Having excluded ventilatory problems and light anaesthesia, a patient displaying these signs should be treated for MH.

The Association of Anaesthetists of Great Britain and Ireland has published guidelines for the recognition and treatment of malignant hyperthermia. These guidelines should be available wherever general anaesthesia is administered, and followed if MH is suspected. Seek senior anaesthetic assistance immediately in all cases of suspected MH.

Discontinue the precipitant, hyperventilate with 100% oxygen and give dantrolene sodium as soon as the diagnosis is considered. The initial dose is 2.5 mg kg^{-1} IV. Repeated doses of 1 mg kg^{-1} are given thereafter to a maximum of 10 mg kg^{-1}. Dantrolene has no major side effects but reconstitution for injection is time-consuming; several people may be needed to help. Further treatment comprises active cooling, treatment of hyperkalaemia, arrhythmias and disseminated intravascular coagulation, frequent monitoring of arterial blood gases, potassium, FBC and clotting, and supportive therapy as required.

Anaphylaxis

Anaphylaxis is a severe, life-threatening, generalized or systemic hypersensitivity reaction. It is characterized by rapidly developing, life-threatening problems involving: the airway (pharyngeal or laryngeal oedema), and/or breathing (bronchospasm with tachypnoea), and/or circulation (hypotension and/or tachycardia). In most cases, there are associated skin and mucosal changes. Almost any drug has the potential to cause anaphylaxis. Other causes include contact with substances such as chlorhexidine, or less commonly, latex.

The clinical manifestations vary, but in the anaesthetized patient the incidences of various signs are:

- cardiovascular collapse 88%;
- erythema 45%;
- bronchospasm 36%;
- angio-oedema 24%;
- other cutaneous signs (swelling, urticaria, rash).

Anaphylaxis on induction will frequently present with acute cardiovascular collapse. The presence of severe bronchospasm may make ventilation of the lungs impossible, and acute upper airway oedema makes intubation difficult. In this situation a smaller tracheal tube or even a surgical airway may be necessary as other rescue devices such as the laryngeal mask airway will be relatively ineffective. An alternative cause of hypotension, high inspiratory pressures and desaturation of arterial blood is tension pneumothorax, particularly in the trauma patient. If there is any doubt about the diagnosis, treat both conditions. Other diagnoses to consider are asthma, airway obstruction and primary myocardial pathology.

The initial treatment of anaphylaxis is to remove the precipitant and to manage the airway, breathing and circulation:

- stop drug/remove precipitant;
- 100% oxygen;
- maintain airway;
- get help;
- lay patient flat with legs elevated;
- adrenaline IV:

  - 50 mcg (0.5 mL of 1:10,000) increments (observing cardiac monitor) every 30 seconds until hypotension/bronchospasm improve;
  - 100 – 500 mcg or more may be required;
  - 1 mcg kg^{-1} in children = 0.1 mL kg^{-1} of 1:100,000;
  - In severe cases consider an adrenaline infusion: the usual dose is 0.05–0.1 mcg kg^{-1} min^{-1};
- IV fluids – crystalloid (20 mL kg^{-1} in children).

Give antihistamines and corticosteroids to treat the end organ response to the mediators. A catecholamine infusion may be required as cardiovascular instability may last for hours. Check arterial blood gases regularly. Bronchodilators may be required to treat persistent bronchospasm. Before attempting extubation, ensure there is no residual oedema by deflating the tracheal tube cuff and checking for an adequate air leak.

- Antihistamines: chlorphenamine 10 – 20 mg slowly IV (0.25 mg kg^{-1} in children);
- Corticosteroids: hydrocortisone 100 – 300 mg IV (4 mg kg^{-1} in children).

The Association of Anaesthetists of Great Britain and Ireland has published guidelines for the recognition and treatment of anaphylaxis. These guidelines should be available wherever general anaesthesia is administered, and followed if anaphylaxis is suspected. Immediately seek senior assistance in all cases of suspected anaphylaxis.

Summary

- Knowledge of the pharmacology and side effects of drugs used commonly in emergency airway management is essential.
- No drug is perfect, and its advantages and disadvantages must be understood clearly.
- Practitioners should choose drugs with which they are most familiar.
- Practitioners must know how to treat the common complications of any drugs or techniques used.

Acknowledgement

This chapter has been updated from the first edition chapter, which was written by Neil Nichol, Nikki Maran and Jonathan Benger.

Further Reading

1   British Medical Association and the Royal Pharmaceutical Society of Great Britain. (2013) *National Formulary*, Number 66. London: British Medical Association and the Royal Pharmaceutical Society of Great Britain.

2   Peck, T.E., Hill, S.A., Williams, M., Grice, A.S., Aldington, D.S. (2003) *Pharmacology for Anaesthesia and Intensive Care*, 2nd edn. London: Greenwich Medical Media.

3   Association of Anaesthetists of Great Britain and Ireland. (2004) Syringe labelling in critical care area (June 2004 update). London: Association of Anaesthetists of Great Britain and Ireland. Available at: http://www.aagbi.org/sites/default/files/SYRINGE%20LABELLING%202014.pdf (accessed November 2014).

4   Association of Anaesthetists of Great Britain and Ireland. (2009) Management of a patient with suspected anaphylaxis during anaesthesia (revised 2009). London: Association of Anaesthetists of Great Britain and Ireland. Available at: http://www.aagbi.org/sites/default/files/ana_laminate_2009.pdf (accessed November 2014).

5   Soar, J., Pumphrey, R., Cant, A. *et al.* (2008) Emergency treatment of anaphylactic reactions – guidelines for healthcare providers. Resuscitation; 77: 157–69.

6   Chan, C.M., Mitchell, A.L., Shorr, A.F. (2012) Etomidate is associated with mortality and adrenal insufficiency in sepsis: a meta-analysis. Crit Care Med; 40: 2945–53.

7   Sunshine, J.E., Deem, S., Weiss, N.S. *et al.* (2013) Etomidate, adrenal function and mortality in critically ill patients. Respir Care; 58: 639–46.

8 Hunter, B.R., Kirschner, J. (2013) In patients with severe sepsis, does a single dose of etomidate to facilitate intubation increase mortality? Ann Emerg Med; 61: 571–2.

9 Cooper, G.M. (2002) Chapter 43: The elderly patient. In Hutton, P. (ed.), *Fundamental Principles and Practice of Anaesthesia*. London: Martin Dunitz Ltd.

10 Rose, M., Fisher, M. Rocuronium: high risk for anaphylaxis? Br J Anaesth 2001; 86: 678–82.

11 Association of Anaesthetists of Great Britain and Ireland. (2011) Malignant Hyperthermia Crisis AAGBI Safety Guideline. Available at: http://www.aagbi.org/sites/default/files/MH_paediatric_laminate_2013_for_members.pdf (accessed November 2014).

12 Curtis, R., Lomax, S., Patel, B. (2012) Use of sugammadex in a 'Can't intubate, can't ventilate' situation. Br J Anaesth; 108: 612–14.

13 Jeevendra Martyn, J.A., Richtsfeld, M. (2006) Succinylcholine-induced hyperkalemia in acquired pathologic states. Anesthesiology; 104: 158–69.

Chapter

8

Rapid sequence induction and tracheal intubation

Jonathan Hulme and Dinendra S. Gill

Objectives

The objectives of this chapter are to:

- Understand the importance of pre-oxygenation.
- Be able to describe the technique of rapid sequence induction of anaesthesia and tracheal intubation.
- Understand how to confirm successful intubation.

Introduction

Rapid sequence induction of anaesthesia (RSI) involves injecting an anaesthetic induction drug to achieve hypnosis, immediately followed by a neuromuscular blocking drug to produce complete paralysis. The lungs are not usually ventilated between induction and intubation to prevent inflation of the stomach. The time from loss of consciousness to securing the airway is minimized because the patient's stomach is assumed to be full.

Preparation

The acutely ill patient is prone to physiological decompensation following emergency anaesthesia, and optimal preparation is essential to minimize this risk.

Preparation for RSI (Chapter 6) requires preparation of the patient, team, equipment, environment and a plan for failure.

This chapter assumes the presence of a trained team, equipment for initial and failed intubation strategies, a standardized RSI checklist (see Appendix 3 for an example) and appropriate patient monitoring.

Emergency Airway Management, Second Edition, ed. Andrew Burtenshaw, Jonathan Benger and Jerry Nolan. Published by Cambridge University Press. © College of Emergency Medicine, London, 2015.

Pre-oxygenation

Effective pre-oxygenation greatly increases the oxygen reserve within the lungs by replacing nitrogen in the alveoli with oxygen. This maximizes the time before desaturation of arterial blood occurs during apnoea, and decreases the risk of severe hypoxaemia and its associated morbidity and mortality.

The time to desaturation is related not only to the effectiveness of pre-oxygenation, but also the body habitus, positioning and physiological state of the patient.

Breathing 100% oxygen with normal tidal volumes and an adequate respiratory rate for 3 minutes before induction of anaesthesia is sufficient for most patients. Use a 20° head-up tilt (reverse Trendelenburg position) whenever possible – this increases the time before desaturation occurs and may also reduce the risk of passive regurgitation of gastric contents.

Some ill patients are not adequately pre-oxygenated with this technique and those with significant lung disease may remain hypoxaemic. A good airway management technique with a well-fitting mask and high-flow oxygen is essential. Gentle application (maximum 10 cmH$_2$O) of positive end expiratory pressure (PEEP) may augment pre-oxygenation in patients failing to achieve an arterial blood oxygen saturation above 95%; avoid inflating the stomach, which causes regurgitation of gastric contents with the risk of aspiration. A patient with a low respiratory rate may not achieve sufficient alveolar ventilation to replace nitrogen in the lungs with oxygen and will require assisted ventilation to achieve adequate pre-oxygenation before RSI.

It is not standard practice to assist ventilation during the period of apnoea between drug delivery and tracheal intubation. However, if the patient required assisted ventilation before induction, continue this after the induction drug has been given while awaiting the onset of complete neuromuscular blockade. Assist ventilation using low tidal volumes, low inflation pressures and a slow rate – this strategy will minimize the risk of gastric insufflation.

Critically ill patients may be agitated for numerous reasons. This may pose a risk to to the patient, as delivery of care, including effective pre-oxygenation, is made more difficult. Injection of small boluses of a sedative drug, typically the same induction drug that will be used for the emergency anaesthesia, titrated to achieve patient compliance, enables better preparation for the procedure and improved pre-oxygenation. Proceeding immediately to anaesthesia and paralysis to treat agitation, thereby foregoing optimization of pre-oxygenation, is unacceptable because of the risk of hypoxaemia and associated harm.

The shape of the oxyhaemoglobin dissociation curve (Figure 2.10) indicates that the rate of decline of oxygen saturation is greatest below 92%; once pulse oximetry indicates a S_pO_2 of 92% or less, ventilate the patient's lungs immediately with 100% oxygen. Ensure that one team member has a nominated role to watch the monitors and is empowered to alert the team to worsening vital signs (e.g. oxygen saturation and blood pressure). Careful preparation and optimal oxygenation are essential before commencing emergency anaesthesia.

Apnoeic oxygenation

Delivery of oxygen to the alveoli is required to prevent arterial blood oxygen desaturation. This is achieved by either spontaneous or assisted ventilation, but after injection of anaesthetic induction and paralyzing drugs, ventilatory effort and delivery of oxygen ceases.

Apnoeic oxygenation continues delivery of oxygen in the absence of ventilation, providing the airway is patent. It increases significantly the time before desaturation of arterial blood occurs during anaesthesia.

Nasal cannulae are sited under the facemask during pre-oxygenation. High-flow oxygen through conventional nasal cannulae can be uncomfortable in conscious patients; increase the oxygen flow from 4 to 15 L min^{-1} at the onset of anaesthesia. High flow nasal oxygenation can slow the desaturation process by improving the oxygen concentration in the proximal divisions of the respiratory tract. This technique is a useful adjunct to formal pre-oxygenation in patients at increased risk of hypoxaemia during induction, or where difficulty with intubation is anticipated. However, if the nasal cannulae tubing prevents an adequate seal being formed this may be counterproductive since it will diminish the benefit of pre-oxygenation, and it should be abandoned.

The technique of rapid sequence induction

Adequate preparation will have been completed (acronym PEACH: see Chapter 6), culminating in a team brief completed using a standardized emergency anaesthesia checklist (see Appendix 3).

Injection of pre-calculated doses of induction and neuromuscular blocking drugs produces unconsciousness and complete paralysis. Both drugs are injected rapidly into a functioning intravenous line with an infusion running to expedite drug delivery.

Cricoid pressure

Cricoid pressure is applied in an attempt to reduce passive reflux of gastric contents into the pharynx and subsequent aspiration into the lungs. Do not apply cricoid pressure in the presence of active vomiting because it may cause oesophageal rupture.

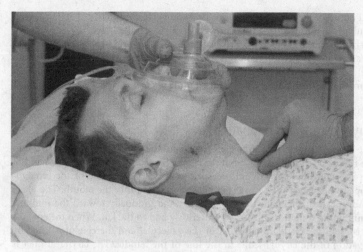

Figure 8.1 Application of cricoid pressure.

The cricoid ring is identified (below the thyroid cartilage and cricothyroid membrane) by a trained assistant and stabilized between the thumb and middle finger before induction of anaesthesia. As consciousness is lost, firm pressure is applied to the centre of the cricoid cartilage using the index finger, pressing directly backwards to compress the upper oesophagus between the cricoid and the cervical vertebra posteriorly (Figure 8.1).

The optimal force is 30–40 newtons, which is enough to be painful in a conscious patient, although how this is judged in the unconscious patient is a significant practical problem (30 newtons is equivalent to the force required to hold a mass of 3 kilograms against gravity). Inadequate pressure will not occlude the oesophagus; however, excessive force or incorrect placement will deform the larynx and make laryngoscopy and intubation more difficult (see Chapter 9). Cricoid pressure is removed only on the instruction of the intubating clinician once correct tube placement has been confirmed, or if it is thought to be distorting the anatomy of the laryngeal inlet and contributing to intubation failure.

The technique of cricoid pressure in clinical practice varies widely, including finger positioning and pressure administered. There is no evidence that a second hand applied behind the neck in an attempt to restrict cervical spine movement is any safer than the standard technique. There is little evidence that use of this common-sense manoeuvre reduces airway soiling or associated harm during induction of anaesthesia and intubation. Therefore, whilst cricoid pressure is a routine part of every emergency RSI and intubation, ease the pressure or remove it completely if it is making intubation more difficult; securing the airway takes absolute precedence over reducing the theoretical risk of regurgitation and aspiration. If cricoid pressure is reduced or removed during an intubation attempt, and before the airway is secured, do this under direct vision and with suction immediately to hand in case regurgitation occurs.

Laryngoscopy and intubation

The laryngoscope is held in the left hand, and the tip of the blade inserted into the right side of the patient's mouth. It may be necessary to adjust the hand of the assistant applying cricoid pressure to enable the handle of the laryngoscope to be placed correctly as the blade is inserted into the mouth. The blade is advanced further into the oropharynx, and gradually toward the midline, maintaining tongue displacement anteriorly and to the left. When the epiglottis is seen, the blade tip is placed in the vallecula, and the epiglottis lifted by elevation of the laryngoscope in the line of the handle. The laryngeal inlet is seen anterior to the arytenoid cartilages, and the vocal cords identified. Suction may be required to improve the view. Identifying the tip of the epiglottis is key to this process, and is sought specifically at each intubation attempt. Levering the handle of the laryngoscope backwards will damage the teeth or soft tissues of the mouth, and will not improve the view (Figure 8.2).

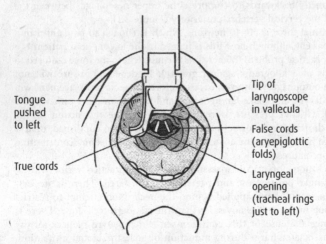

Figure 8.2 The optimal view during laryngoscopy.

The laryngeal view is classified according to the Cormack and Lehane grading system (Figure 5.1).

Use suction to clear any secretions, blood or vomit before passing the tracheal tube through the cords under direct vision.

Routine use of a size 4 laryngoscope blade (for adults) and an intubating bougie is recommended during RSI, and increases the likelihood of successful intubation. The tip of the bougie is bent to form an elbow (coudé), shaped like a hockey stick. With the laryngoscope in place, the bougie is passed behind the epiglottis and into the trachea. Detection of clicks as the bougie slides over the tracheal rings helps to confirm correct placement. DO NOT push the bougie further to wedge in the distal airways. Whilst this may provide secondary confirmation of placement it can also cause an airway injury or pneumothorax.

While the practitioner maintains the best possible view of the larynx the tracheal tube is then railroaded over the bougie into the trachea: this requires the tracheal tube to be threaded over the bougie by an assistant until they are able to grasp the end of the bougie as it protrudes from the tracheal tube. Whilst the bougie is held still, the practitioner advances the tracheal tube over the bougie under direct vision. Rotation of the tracheal tube 90° counter-clockwise may ease passage through the cords. While grasping the tracheal tube firmly, the assistant removes the bougie and correct placement is confirmed using the methods described below. Both the practitioner and assistant must be trained and practised in the use of a bougie. Common errors include advancing the tube into the trachea before the assistant has grasped the free end of the bougie, failure to maintain the best possible laryngeal view whilst railroading the tracheal tube and failure to rotate the tracheal tube as it passes the cords.

Some practitioners use an intubating stylet, a stiff but malleable introducer inserted into, but not protruding beyond the distal tip of, the tracheal tube. The tube can be preformed into a J shape to facilitate manipulation through the cords.

During intubation, if the laryngeal inlet and vocal cords cannot be seen immediately, the following interventions may improve the grade of view:

- Ensure optimal positioning of the patient and practitioner.
- Backward, upward and rightward pressure (BURP) on the larynx by an assistant may improve the view. The BURP manoeuvre is different to cricoid pressure.
- Use an alternative laryngoscope. This may be a variant of a standard blade (e.g. McCoy blade) or a videolaryngoscope that is not reliant on an unobstructed straight-line view from the mouth to the larynx to see the cords. A videolaryngoscope is an example of an optical laryngoscope, although other devices are also available.
- Reduce or release cricoid pressure. Continue laryngoscopy while this is done so the effect on the view can be seen and to detect immediately any regurgitation of gastric contents.

During emergency anaesthesia, a failed intubation is declared after a maximum of three intubation attempts.

If difficulty is encountered, ask for help immediately and consider whether waking the patient up is a viable option if intubation is unsuccessful. Have a clear plan for failure before commencing RSI, including formal consideration of whether waking the patient is an option. Communicate this plan clearly to the team in advance.

Videolaryngoscopy

The introduction of video laryngoscopes, either as part of standard laryngoscopy or when managing a difficult airway, may transform the approach to RSI. There are several designs available, but in most a minaturized video camera or optical system allows a view 'round the corner', particularly when the larynx is anteriorly placed or when neck immobilization or limited movement prevents optimal positioning. It is rare not to achieve a view at least as good as that obtained with conventional laryngoscopy and often the view is at least one Cormack and Lehane grade better. When documenting the grade of intubation, be specific about whether the view of the cords described is via a videolaryngoscope or by direct laryngoscopy. (Cormack and Lehane descriptions refer traditionally to direct view.) Even when a videolaryngoscope has been used it is good practice to record the direct view intubation grade to facilitate decision-making if intubation is required in the future.

Depending on the type, video laryngoscopes are used like a standard laryngoscope or with a modified approach. For most devices only short periods of manikin or clinical training are required to achieve optimal views consistently.

Although the larynx is generally easier to see, intubation can be more difficult, particularly when more acutely curved blades are used. This may be overcome by increased clinical experience, use of a bougie, malleable stylets or alternative designs of tracheal tubes. Several devices have integrated tube guides to reduce this problem.

Confirmation of tracheal tube placement

Once placed correctly in the trachea, the tracheal tube is advanced until the cuff lies just beyond the vocal cords, and the cuff is then inflated slowly until there is no air leak during lung inflation. Ideally a pressure gauge is used to ensure the correct cuff pressure. On some tracheal tubes correct depth is facilitated by the presence of a black line just above the cuff, which should be located at the level of the cords. As a general rule, it is to be expected that when the tracheal tube is at the correct depth the patient's teeth will lie between 20 and 21 cm in an adult female and 22 and 23 cm in an adult male. Correct placement of the tube is confirmed using the following methods.

Carbon dioxide detection is the gold standard by which placement of the tracheal tube in the airway is confirmed: it must be undertaken routinely, using waveform capnography. In remote locations, a disposable colourimetric CO_2 detector may be useful to confirm tube placement on the first breath, but does not replace the need for waveform capnography. The following additional checks are carried out by attaching the breathing system to the tracheal tube and ventilating the patient's lungs manually, but alone do not confirm correct tube placement:

- Inspect the chest wall looking for symmetry of movement with ventilation.
- Use a stethoscope to listen in both axillae for air entry, and listen in the epigastrium to confirm absence of air insufflating the stomach.

Once tracheal intubation is confirmed, release the cricoid pressure and secure the tube. Ribbon tie is used typically, but proprietary tube holder devices are also available. In a patient with raised intracranial pressure use of adhesive tape instead of a tie will avoid compression of the jugular veins, which has the potential to impair venous drainage and increase intracranial pressure. However, this theoretical risk must be weighed against the possibility of tube displacement as the patient is transported around the hospital or to another hospital. It is not good practice to insert an oropharyngeal airway adjacent to the tracheal tube. These airway adjuncts are not intended as bite blocks and have been associated with dental damage and intra-oral pressure damage. Waveform capnography must be used wherever RSI is undertaken.

Post-intubation review

The patient is now reassessed, with specific evaluation of the airway, ventilation and circulation. Inject a long-acting neuromuscular blocking drug if indicated. Use a suction catheter to clear material from the proximal airways. Check the monitors for heart rate, S_pO_2, blood pressure, end tidal CO_2 and peak inspiratory pressure. Request a chest X-ray; it is the responsibility of the intubating clinician to examine the chest film, check the position of the tube and to withdraw or advance the tracheal tube as required.

The stages of rapid sequence induction of anaesthesia and tracheal intubation are shown in Figure 8.3.

Summary

- Successful completion of rapid sequence induction and tracheal intubation depends on careful preparation and attention to each stage, with effective use of the team as a resource.
- Optimal pre-oxygenation decreases morbidity and mortality; there are several strategies required to achieve this, including head-up positioning,

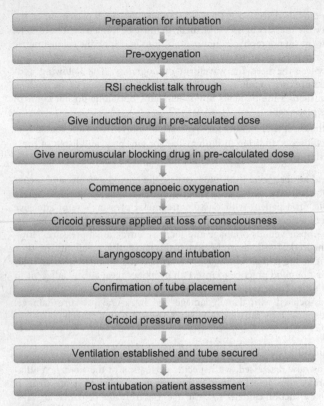

Figure 8.3 The stages of rapid sequence induction of anaesthesia.

administration of a high concentration of oxygen via a well-fitting face mask with or without PEEP and apnoeic oxygenation.

- Before embarking on this procedure the practitioner must have a plan for failed intubation that has been articulated clearly to the team.

Acknowledgement

This chapter has been updated from the first edition chapter, which was written by Neil Nichol, Nikki Maran and Simon Leigh-Smith.

Further reading

1   Association of Anaesthetists of Great Britain and Ireland. (2007) Recommendations for standards of monitoring during anaesthesia and recovery (4th edition) (also appenda published 2011). Available at: http://www.aagbi.org/sites/default/files/standardsofmonitoring07.pdf (accessed November 2014).

2   Weingart, S.D., Levitan, R.M. (2012) Preoxygenation and prevention of desaturation during emergency airway management. Ann Emerg Med; 59: 165–75.

3   Ellis, D.Y., Harris, T., Zideman, D. (2007) Cricoid pressure in emergency department rapid sequence tracheal intubations: a risk-benefit analysis. Ann Emerg Med; 50: 653–65.

4   The Royal College of Anaesthetists and the Difficult Airway Society. (2011) Fourth National Audit Project of the Royal College of Anaesthetists: Major complications of airway management in the UK. Available at: http://www.rcoa.ac.uk/nap4 (accessed November 2014).

Difficult and failed airway

Dermot McKeown and Gavin Lloyd

Objectives

The objectives of this chapter are to:

- Understand the critical importance of maintaining oxygenation after failed intubation following rapid sequence induction (RSI).
- Describe a plan for control of the airway and oxygenation after failed intubation.
- Understand the common causes of failure to obtain an adequate view of the larynx and describe ways of improving the view.
- Understand the reasons for failure to intubate the trachea, and describe techniques that may improve success.
- Understand the techniques for rescue ventilation of the lungs.

At the conclusion of a planned RSI, failure to detect expired CO_2 indicates incorrect placement of the tracheal tube: under these circumstances the tube must be removed. Failure to place a tracheal tube correctly after an RSI is not a disaster, but failure to recognize incorrect placement, or to allow the patient to become injured during further attempts to secure an airway, are indefensible.

> If in doubt, take it out.

Failed first attempt at tracheal intubation during RSI

This situation demands a logical sequence of treatment decisions: the urgency will be dictated by the rate of deterioration in the patient's physiology, which must be considered continuously during further treatment.

Emergency Airway Management, Second Edition, ed. Andrew Burtenshaw, Jonathan Benger and Jerry Nolan. Published by Cambridge University Press. © College of Emergency Medicine, London, 2015.

The fundamental questions are:

- Is the patient's arterial blood oxygenated sufficiently to enable further attempts at intubation safely?
- If not, can it be improved?
- Were the intubating conditions ideal?
- Can the laryngeal view be improved?
- Can the intubation technique be improved?
- Should further attempts fail, are there suitable alternatives?
- Should further attempts fail, is a surgical airway necessary and possible?

Ensuring oxygenation

The Difficult Airway Society guidelines recommend a maximum of three attempts at intubation. However, during airway interventions, pay constant attention to maintaining adequate arterial blood oxygen saturation (S_pO_2). No absolute rules for timing can be given, as the reserves of oxygen available to individual patients are variable: a previously fit young patient with a primary neurological problem, such as an isolated head injury, who has been carefully pre-oxygenated using a well-fitting facemask, is likely to maintain good S_pO_2 values during further intubation attempts; the arterial blood of an obese patient with pulmonary contusions or pneumonia will desaturate rapidly without active ventilation with supplementary oxygen.

Patients need oxygen, not a tube.

Continuous S_pO_2 monitoring is essential. Cease intubation attempts and reoxygenate the patient's lungs before the decrease in S_pO_2 reaches the steep part of the oxyhaemoglobin dissociation curve: this point is 92%. Delegate a member of the team to state when this point has been reached so that the practitioner can stop the intubation attempt and reoxygenate the patient's lungs. When oxygenation failure is a major feature prompting intubation, these conditions may not be achievable, but critical desaturation should be avoided where possible.

Oxygenation techniques

If the airway is clear, apnoeic oxygenation, as described in Chapter 8, may assist in delaying arterial blood desaturation. If the patient is still paralyzed, bag-mask ventilation as described earlier is the first choice (see Chapter 3). Maintain cricoid pressure initially, but if ventilation proves difficult, reduce or release it under direct vision. Improvement in oxygenation is the main goal; this should be achieved easily if ventilation is efficient; even small volumes of high concentrations of oxygen can improve S_pO_2 dramatically. At this stage effective oxygenation has priority over optimal ventilation and CO_2 removal.

Two practitioners are required to optimize ventilation using a bag-mask: one to hold the mask and continue airway manipulations and the other to ventilate the patient's lungs. Ideally, the second individual should also be experienced in airway management and ventilation. Use oropharyngeal and/ or nasopharyngeal airways as necessary to improve airway patency.

If the S_pO_2 continues to decrease despite optimal attempts at bag-mask ventilation, the first rescue technique of choice is to insert a supraglottic airway device (SAD), such as a second generation laryngeal mask airway (LMA); all practitioners attempting intubation must be familiar with these devices. A technique of insertion is described below. Many versions of SADs are available but 'second generation' SADs such as the i-gel™ or ProSeal™ LMA (PLMA) are now widely available, and have advantages for assisted ventilation, which are described below.

Use of a supraglottic airway device (SAD)

SADs have transformed the airway management of patients undergoing elective surgery. If used correctly, they provide an excellent airway for the spontaneously breathing patient and can also be used for controlled ventilation (Figure 9.1).

While it does not provide a cuffed tube in the trachea, and therefore is not considered a 'definitive airway', some degree of protection is afforded since a correctly placed SAD sits in the upper oesophagus and partially protects the glottic opening.

SADs have also been used widely in emergency airway management. As rescue devices, successful insertion rates are high and they have several advantages over other failed airway techniques. Insertion skills are at least as easy to teach as for other devices, and are retained well.

The SAD is recommended as the rescue device of choice in the anaesthetic 'can't intubate, can't oxygenate' (CICO) situation.

Second generation developments of the classic LMA include the PLMA, which enables higher inflation pressures, drainage of the stomach via an oesophageal lumen, and probably greater protection against aspiration (Figure 9.2), the intubating laryngeal mask airway (ILMA), which enables blind passage of a specially designed tracheal tube and the i-gel (Figure 9.1). Blind intubation through the ILMA requires considerable practice before it can be achieved with consistently high success rates. The i-gel has a non-inflatable cuff, oesophageal drainage lumen and integral bite-block. The i-gel is used widely during cardiopulmonary resuscitation, particularly when a practitioner skilled in tracheal intubation is not immediately available.

The recommended technique of insertion for each of these varies slightly from the original LMA.

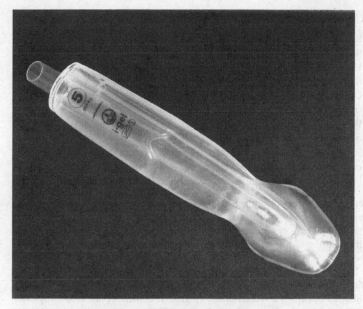

Figure 9.1 An example of a supraglottic airway device.

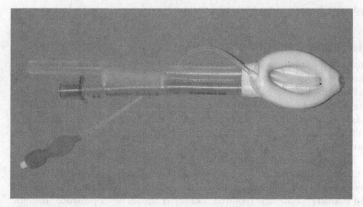

Figure 9.2 The ProSeal laryngeal mask airway.

Technique of insertion of an i-gel SAD

- Remove the device from its packaging and protective cradle and lubricate the back, front and sides of the cuff.
- Unless contra-indicated, place the head and neck in the 'sniffing the morning air' intubation position.
- Open the mouth with a 'scissor' grip (in which the fingers and thumb cross), lifting the chin forward.
- Press the i-gel against the hard palate, and guide it along the posterior oropharynx until definitive resistance is felt.
- Release the cricoid pressure during insertion to enable the i-gel to sit correctly in the upper oesophagus.
- Fix the device in position with self-adhesive tape round the tube.

There are a number of other SADs available for which the relevant manufacturers' insertion instructions should be referred to before use.

If spontaneous respiratory effort resumes, synchronize assisted ventilation with breathing to minimize leakage of gas from the larynx and risk of gastric distension.

Insertion of the SAD is usually easy, and improvement in ventilation rapid. Failure to achieve adequate ventilation may be caused by laryngospasm or obstruction from a folded-down epiglottis. If there is not rapid improvement, make a second attempt to place the SAD. Avoid repeated attempts at insertion if the patient's condition is deteriorating. If oxygenation cannot be maintained with an optimally placed SAD, a surgical approach to the airway is indicated (see below). Although this is a rare event, delay in recognizing the need for a surgical airway can be lethal.

Intubating conditions

Attempting intubation in the presence of muscle tone will cause problems: either failure to see the larynx because of gagging, or failure to pass the tracheal tube because of cord closure. Do not attempt laryngoscopy until the muscle relaxant is fully effective; for suxamethonium this is after the fasciculations have stopped. Loss of jaw tone will indicate the onset of relaxation. If conditions are not optimal, maintain oxygenation while awaiting muscle relaxation.

Manipulation of the tube can be difficult if it is soft (more likely if stored in warm conditions), or flexible because of small calibre. A malleable stylet may enable more efficient direction of the tube, but it will have to be removed if an intubating bougie is required. The stylet should never protrude from the distal end of the tracheal tube.

Do not use a tracheal tube that is too large for the larynx: it will make intubation much more difficult and may cause mucosal pressure damage. Ensure immediate availability of a tube one or two sizes smaller, and the presence of skilled, dedicated assistance for the practitioner undertaking airway management.

Can the laryngeal view be improved?

A full and clear view of the larynx will usually enable an 'easy' intubation; however, a single upper peg tooth can make placement of the tracheal tube difficult despite a good view and, very rarely, the patient may have an airway stenosis beyond the glottis. If the view at first attempt has been partially or totally obscured, there are several techniques that may improve the view. If preparation has been performed carefully, the first attempt should be the best.

Always make the first attempt the best attempt.

Improve the view by clearing secretions, blood and debris rapidly with a wide-bore suction device, followed by one or more of:

- head elevation;
- external manipulation of the larynx;
- use of an alternative laryngoscope or blade, including videolaryngoscopy;
- change of practitioner.

Head elevation

Optimal positioning should have been achieved before the first attempt, but ensure that the head is extended fully at the atlanto-occipital joint and the neck is flexed. These manoeuvres cannot be applied to a patient whose cervical spine is stabilized. Hospital trolleys rarely have an adjustable head support, so insertion of a second pillow or doubling of the pillow may be necessary. An assistant lifting the head can be a suitable alternative, and may be combined with external manipulation of the larynx.

The obese patient poses considerable challenges, and careful positioning of the head and shoulders will facilitate intubation (see Figures 6.1 and 6.2).

Avoid levering the laryngoscope, and ensure that the blade is lifted in the direction of the handle.

External manipulation of larynx

Manipulation of the larynx during laryngoscopy can improve the view: one technique is the Backwards Upwards Rightwards Pressure (BURP) manoeuvre, which can be applied by an assistant. This is not always the most effective direction of manipulation, and alternatively, bimanual laryngoscopy has also been shown to be effective. In this technique the intubating practitioner initially applies external pressure over the thyroid cartilage with their right hand while simultaneously observing the view during direct laryngoscopy. Once an optimum view is achieved, an assistant maintains this positioning, so that tracheal intubation can proceed. If necessary, the position can be modified during the procedure. Use of a videolaryngoscope with an external monitor enables the assistant to manipulate the larynx to achieve the best view.

Use of an alternative laryngoscope or blade

A Macintosh curved blade laryngoscope is currently the most widely used instrument for tracheal intubation. Familiarity with proper technique, and continued practice, will result in very high rates of successful laryngoscopy and intubation.

The practitioner should select their favoured blade from the outset – this minimizes the likelihood of needing to change the blade, particularly if a large blade is used. It may be reasonable to use the same blade again for a second attempt. Smaller blades may be useful in smaller patients as they provide more 'curve' in the oral cavity during laryngoscopy.

Use of an alternative laryngoscope

If the practitioner is familiar with alternative blade types, for example the McCoy blade (and has maintained skills in their use) it may be appropriate to change the blade once. However, where a videolaryngoscope is available and the practitioner is experienced in its use this will usually be the preferred substitute.

Videolaryngoscopy

Videolaryngoscopy, as described in Chapter 8, is increasingly used as the initial approach in emergencies, and is highly effective, providing the intubating practitioner is suitably skilled and practiced in its use.

Change of practitioner

As with any practical procedure, it is easy to become obsessed with the belief that 'I should successfully intubate this patient' rather than 'this patient should be successfully intubated'. If the first attempt has been the best attempt, and further manipulations have not been successful, another experienced practitioner may consider attempting intubation, but only if it is safe to do so. This must not result in a queue of potential experts performing multiple attempts; however, most series of emergency RSI failures demonstrate that a change of practitioner, particularly to a more experienced one, usually enables successful intubation. A change in practitioner also provides a useful educational opportunity to observe techniques that may prove successful.

This sequence may be conveniently remembered by the mnemonic O HELP! (Box 9.1).

Box 9.1 O HELP!

- **O**xygenation
- **H**ead elevation
- **E**xternal laryngeal manipulation
- **L**aryngoscope or blade change
- **P**al – call for assistance

If the second laryngoscopy fails to improve the view

If the view of the larynx cannot be improved, and oxygenation remains acceptable, an intubating bougie may be useful. Depending on their experience with this device, many practitioners use the intubating bougie at the initial laryngoscopy if the view is grade 2 or 3. This device can be passed into the trachea either anterior to visible arytenoids, where a grade 2 view is obtainable, or posterior to the epiglottis blindly if the view is grade 3. A characteristic 'clicking' sensation may be detected as the angulated tip of the bougie moves over the tracheal rings. It is essential to advance the bougie gently, as excessive force can cause perforation of the airway. If muscle power is returning, there may be coughing or other reaction to tracheal placement of the bougie. Further information on the correct use of an intubating bougie is given in Chapter 8.

Several versions of the intubating bougie exist: the most reliable and preferred device is a coudé-tipped single use tracheal tube introducer.

If repeat laryngoscopy fails, but oxygenation is maintained

In the 'can't intubate, can oxygenate' situation the practitioner must consider the following:

- Is spontaneous breathing present?
- Is ventilation adequate?
- Is the airway still at risk?
- Is intubation the only option at this time?

After a single dose of suxamethonium, in the absence of opioid, by the time that repeat laryngoscopy has been undertaken, intubation has not been achieved, and oxygenation is in progress, neuromuscular function is likely to be recovering and spontaneous breathing resuming. This should prompt synchronization of ventilatory assistance with spontaneous respiration, and a gradual return to the pre-RSI state.

Spontaneous breathing may be inadequate, and assistance may need to be continued to ensure either oxygenation, ventilation or both. Whether or not

---

Box 9.2 Some alternative methods that may be used by expert practitioners

- Videolaryngoscopy
- Intubating laryngeal mask with or without fibreoptic guidance
- Alternative laryngoscopes or optical stylets
- Light-wand techniques
- Fibreoptic laryngoscopy via laryngeal mask with Aintree catheter
- Awake fibreoptic laryngoscopy and intubation
- Retrograde intubation
- Awake intubation with local anaesthesia
- Blind nasal intubation

This list is not comprehensive, and all techniques demand considerable practice to attain mastery.

---

adequate spontaneous breathing has returned will dictate the need for, and urgency of, progression to alternative intubation techniques. A judgement of airway risk should also be made at this time: where oxygenation and ventilation are adequate, and airway patency is maintained, alternatives can be considered calmly; if the airway is deteriorating (e.g. expanding neck haematoma), there is far greater urgency. A choice must be made between continuing the intubation sequence, or accepting that the risk/benefit for this patient at this time is to cease intubation attempts and maintain the airway without intubation. If a 'best' attempt at laryngoscopy and intubation by an experienced practitioner has failed, and review of 'O HELP' has failed, it is unlikely that tracheal intubation will be achieved using standard methods.

Patients do not die from failure to intubate, they die from failure to stop trying to intubate.

This does not preclude further attempts using alternative techniques by experienced airway practitioners. Skills such as fibreoptic methods, retrograde techniques, and use of intubating laryngeal masks or light wands are difficult to acquire and retain, and beyond the remit of this manual (Box 9.2). The best option may be to maintain oxygenation and ventilation with basic techniques until an experienced practitioner arrives.

If repeat laryngoscopy fails, and oxygenation is not maintained

The CICO situation is rare, but a logical plan must be in place to enable difficult decisions to be made rapidly. The first action is to insert a SAD. If oxygenation cannot be maintained with a SAD, consider the following questions:

- **Is a surgical airway necessary?**
- Are the patient's lungs being ventilated maximally with oxygen?
- **Is a surgical airway necessary?**
- Is arterial oxygenation stable and survivable? Can it be improved?
- **Is a surgical airway necessary?**
- Will a surgical airway be possible?
- Which form of surgical airway?

> The ideal rate of cricothyroidotomy is 100% in those who need it, and 0% in those who do not.

Is a surgical airway necessary?

Creating a surgical airway is a rare event. Large case series in the US report cricothyroidotomy rates of 0.5% for emergency department intubations. This is considerably higher than the incidence in the UK and elsewhere in Europe. It is important to consider that a surgical airway may be necessary, and to be prepared to proceed: although early consideration is essential, it may not be mandated immediately.

Are the patient's lungs being ventilated maximally with oxygen?

If the patient's lungs are being ventilated adequately, yet arterial blood oxygenation cannot be maintained at >90% S_pO_2, check that oxygen is being delivered to the correct breathing system and to the patient. Disconnected tubing, failure to turn oxygen on and the use of other gases are all causes of oxygenation failure.

Is a surgical airway necessary?

Although the previous check has been rapid, the situation may be deteriorating. Failure to identify simple causes increases the likely need for a surgical airway.

Is arterial oxygenation stable and survivable? Can it be improved?

The S_pO_2 in relation to the patient's pre-existing condition is important: a stable saturation of 85% in a patient with pulmonary oedema with apparently adequate ventilation may not be increased by intubation alone; application of positive end expiratory pressure (PEEP) or continuous positive airway pressure (CPAP) or non-invasive positive pressure ventilation (CPAP/NIPPV) may slowly increase the S_pO_2.

Stable, survivable oxygenation with no ventilatory difficulty and no impending airway problem is again a situation that may enable more experienced help to be mobilized.

Is a surgical airway necessary?

A surgical airway is indicated if a rapid check has shown no equipment problems and there is failure to oxygenate and oxygenate the lungs.

Will a surgical airway be possible?

This is not the time to consider this. Assessment of the patient before RSI should have identified potential problems for individual patients. At this stage the airway is required, and equipment must be immediately available. The team needs to be prepared and know their roles and responsibilities.

Techniques for rescue ventilation

Failure to intubate combined with failure to oxygenate is an uncommon but time-critical situation, which occurs more commonly in victims of trauma. Rescue devices such as the classic LMA or a second generation SAD will often convert a 'can't oxygenate' situation into a 'can oxygenate' situation. If this fails a surgical airway or needle cricothyroidotomy are required. Published studies of emergency surgical airways demonstrate that, even in this stressful situation, success rates for this procedure are very high. The commonest error is performing the procedure too late, when hypoxaemic damage may have already occurred. There are various techniques that can be used, and many commercial kits are available. Doctors who may be responsible for emergency airway management must be familiar with the equipment in their hospitals and confident in its use. Most doctors will never have to perform a surgical airway, but if required to do so they must perform the procedure rapidly and effectively. The straightforward techniques described below require equipment that should be available in every emergency department.

Surgical cricothyroidotomy provides a definitive airway that can be used to ventilate the lungs until semi-elective intubation or tracheostomy is performed. Needle cricothyroidotomy is a much more temporary intervention providing only short-term oxygenation. It requires a high-pressure oxygen source, may cause barotrauma, particularly in the presence of expiratory obstruction, and can be particularly ineffective in patients with chest trauma. It is also prone to failure because of kinking of the cannula, and is unsuitable for maintaining oxygenation during patient transfer. It is often recommended in the (very rare) failed airway in a child, where surgical cricothyroidotomy is relatively contra-indicated because of the risk of damaging the cricoid cartilage.

The final choice of surgical airway will depend upon the clinical situation, practitioner training, skills and experience. Options are:

- needle cricothyroidotomy;
- surgical cricothyroidotomy;
- tracheostomy.

Needle cricothyroidotomy

Insertion of a wide-bore, non-kinking cannula through the cricothyroid membrane and using this to deliver oxygen can be life-saving. The correct equipment must be available to connect to an oxygen source. This equipment should be identified clearly and stored for immediate use: an emergency is not the time to develop improvized solutions for oxygen delivery.

Experience with bench models of cricothyroid puncture is useful and some practitioners will have experienced insertion of cannulae into the trachea during percutaneous tracheostomy. Effective needle cricothyroidotomy may not provide entirely adequate oxygenation and ventilation, and does not prevent the risk of aspiration, but will usually provide enough oxygenation to enable a more formal airway intervention to proceed.

Equipment required

- stiff cannula and needle (minimum 14 gauge in adults);
- syringe (preferably 20 mL);
- ventilation system that can be attached securely at one end to a high-pressure oxygen source at 400 kPa (4 bar), and at the other to the cannula; this should enable control of inspiration and expiration with effective pressure release.

Technique

- Attach the syringe to the rear of the cannula and needle assembly, and insert the cannula through the cricothyroid membrane into the airway at an angle of 45 degrees, aiming caudally in the midline. Confirm cannula position by aspiration of air with the syringe and advance the cannula fully over the needle into the trachea. Remove the needle, and aspirate air from the cannula to confirm position.
- Hold the cannula in place, attach the ventilation system and commence ventilation.
- One second of oxygen supplied at a pressure of 400 kPa (4 bar) and flow of 15 L min^{-1} should be sufficient to inflate adult lungs adequately. This is followed by a four-second pause to enable expiration via the upper airway (expiration does not occur via the cannula). In children, the initial oxygen

flow rate in L min^{-1} should equal the child's age in years, and this is increased in 1 L min^{-1} increments until one second of oxygen flow causes the chest to rise.

- Look carefully for adequate exhalation through the upper airway. This usually occurs without difficulty, but it is essential to ensure that the chest falls adequately after each ventilation.
- If ventilation fails or complications occur, proceed **immediately** to surgical cricothyroidotomy.

Note: a major problem with this technique is occlusion of the cannula after insertion. This is especially likely where a soft, kinkable intravenous cannula is used. The Fourth National Audit Project (NAP4) report identified an approximately 60% failure rate of emergency cannula cricothyroidotomy, raising the possibility that surgical cricothyroidotomy is superior to needle cricothyroidotomy. The report recommended that surgical cricothyroidotomy should be taught alongside needle cricothyroidotomy.

Surgical cricothyroidotomy

The cricothyroid membrane is relatively avascular and normally easy to feel. Extension of the neck (if possible) will improve surgical access and exposure.

Equipment required

- scalpel (preferably 20 blade: rounded rather than pointed);
- 6 or 7mm cuffed tracheal tube;
- tracheal dilator (artery clip if unavailable);
- intubating bougie.

Technique

- Rapidly but accurately identify the cricothyroid membrane.
- Make a horizontal stab incision through the membrane into the airway.
- Open the incision with tracheal dilators or clip (with the scalpel blade still *in situ*).
- Remove the scalpel blade and insert the intubating bougie into the trachea.
- Railroad the tracheal tube over the intubating bougie to place it in the trachea.
- Inflate the cuff and confirm tube position.

Note: this procedure should be completed in approximately 30 seconds.

Be careful not to damage the posterior tracheal wall by deep penetration with the scalpel blade. If the incision is too small to admit the tube the incision can be enlarged laterally while being held open vertically with the tracheal dilator. Ideally, once a passage is made into the trachea it should be occupied by instruments until a tube is inserted. This technique prevents loss of the passage at a crucial time and minimizes bleeding. A tracheal tube is preferred to a tracheostomy tube because the cuff of a small tracheostomy tube is often too small to occlude an adult trachea.

Tracheostomy

A surgical tracheostomy will rarely be indicated as a primary method of securing the airway. This is a formal surgical procedure that cannot be undertaken safely without training. Percutaneous tracheostomy can be used in emergencies, but only by individuals experienced in the single-stage dilatational approach.

Summary

- A well planned RSI by an experienced practitioner with adequate pre-assessment will have a high success rate for correct placement of a tracheal tube at the first attempt.
- If the tube is not inserted easily, and oxygenation is well maintained, several rapid manipulations may be made in an attempt to improve the laryngeal view and optimize intubating conditions.
- If intubation is still unsuccessful, ensure adequate oxygenation before a second laryngoscopy and intubation sequence. This attempt may include repositioning, external laryngeal manipulation, and a change of equipment or practitioner. An intubating bougie will frequently be used to assist intubation with reduced view (grade 2 or 3).
- Failure to intubate again must be followed by reoxygenation/ventilation, and a reassessment of the need and urgency for intubation.
- The rescue technique of choice is bag-mask ventilation but if this fails insert a supraglottic airway device.
- Adequate oxygenation and ventilation and a stable airway at this point will enable careful consideration of a different approach by a practitioner with specialist airway skills.
- Continued failure to oxygenate mandates rapid checks for remediable causes.
- If oxygenation continues to deteriorate, a surgical airway is indicated. The method chosen will depend on patient and practitioner factors, but a surgical technique is preferred over needle cricothyroidotomy in adults if the practitioner has this skill.

Acknowledgement

This chapter has been updated from the first edition chapter, which was written by Dermot McKeown, Tim Parke and David Lockey.

Further reading

1 Henderson, J.J., Popat, M.T., Latto, I.P., Pearce, A.C. (2004) Difficult Airway Society guidelines for management of the unanticipated difficult intubation. Anaesthesia; 59: 675–94.

2 American Society of Anesthesiologists Task Force on Management of the Difficult Airway. (2013) Practice guidelines for management of the difficult airway: an updated report by the American Society of Anesthesiologists Task Force on Management of the Difficult Airway. Anesthesiology; 118: 251–70.

3 Levitan, R.M. (2003) Patient safety in emergency airway management and rapid sequence intubation: metaphorical lessons from skydiving. Ann Emerg Med; 42: 81–7.

4 Murphy, M.F. (2003) Bringing the larynx into view: a piece of the puzzle. Ann Emerg Med; 41: 338–41.

5 Levitan, R.M., Kinkle, W.C., Levin, W.J., Everett, W.W. (2006) Laryngeal view during laryngoscopy: a randomised trial comparing cricoid pressure, backward-upward-rightward pressure, and bimanual laryngoscopy. Ann Emerg Med; 47: 548–55.

6 Bair, A.E., Panacek, E.A., Wisner, D.H., Bales, R., Sakles, J.C. (2003) Cricothyrotomy: a 5-year experience at one institution. J Emerg Med; 24: 151–6.

7 Hamaekers, A.E., Henderson, J.J. (2011) Equipment and strategies for emergency tracheal access in the adult patient. Anaesthesia; 66: 65–80.

8 The Difficult Airway Society of the United Kingdom. Website and algorithms are available at: www.das.uk.com (accessed November 2014).

9 The Royal College of Anaesthetists and The Difficult Airway Society. (2011) *NAP4. Fourth National Audit Project of The Royal College of Anaesthetists and The Difficult Airway Society. Major complications of airway management in the United Kingdom.* ISBN 978-1-900936-03-3.

Chapter 10

Post-intubation management

Paul Younge and John C. Berridge

Objectives

The objectives of this chapter are to:

- Understand the principles of patient management following successful intubation.
- Understand the principles of monitoring, sedation and neuromuscular blockade for intubated patients.
- Be familiar with the correct operation of transport ventilators.
- Be familiar with the principles of patient preparation for safe transfer.

Introduction

After RSI and tracheal intubation has been achieved successfully there is often an understandable sense of relief that the airway has been secured. However, intubation is only the initial phase of management; the post-intubation phase is equally important.

Following emergency airway management, most patients will need transfer to other areas such as the radiology department, intensive care unit (ICU), operating room or tertiary care in another hospital. The key questions are:

- What is the predicted clinical course?
- Is the patient stable enough to transfer?
- Is any further treatment required?
- What measures are required for safe transfer?

The objectives of the post-intubation phase are to achieve enough physiological stability for transfer, and to carry out other appropriate treatment.

Emergency Airway Management, Second Edition, ed. Andrew Burtenshaw, Jonathan Benger and Jerry Nolan. Published by Cambridge University Press. © College of Emergency Medicine, London, 2015.

The requirements for stabilization and the nature of treatment may vary considerably; for example, a patient intubated for overdose can often be stabilized and treated while waiting for an ICU bed. A patient with a suspected traumatic extradural haemorrhage should undergo CT scanning as soon as adequate physiological stability is achieved. An unstable multiple-trauma patient may need urgent transfer to the operating room to achieve surgical haemorrhage control. The increasing importance of CT results to guide trauma management has resulted in an increasing need to transfer unstable patients to the scanner. These transfers and decisions can be challenging.

This phase can be described using a modified ABCDE system. The sections below form a checklist. While an ABCDE system suggests progress in a consecutive manner, procedures will normally be carried out simultaneously when a team is involved.

Airway

Is the airway secure?

Secure the tracheal tube at the correct length with a tie or tape to avoid unplanned extubation, or intubation of the right main bronchus. There are many methods of securing a tracheal tube: choose one that is safe, effective, and familiar. A common method for tying the tube is shown in Figure 10.1.

Tape is sometimes preferred in the setting of head injury to avoid encircling the neck and impeding venous return, which may increase intracranial pressure. Several commercial fixation devices are also available. These are effective but rather more expensive than the conventional alternatives.

Has end tidal CO_2 monitoring been attached?

Continuous waveform end tidal carbon-dioxide (E_TCO_2) measurement is essential and, as well as confirmation of ongoing correct tube placement, it enables monitoring of alveolar ventilation and respiratory pattern. It is particularly important in the setting of head injury where precise control of P_aCO_2 is required. Record the E_TCO_2 at the time an arterial blood sample is taken: this enables calibration of the E_TCO_2 against P_aCO_2. The latter may be significantly higher because of $\dot{V}/\dot{Q}$ mismatch.

Is the cervical spine adequately stabilized?

Is an HME filter (heat and moisture exchange) at the patient end of the circuit?

Apart from protecting equipment from contamination this will help keep the patient warm and maintain airway humidification. This prevents excessive drying of secretions and reduces the likelihood of respiratory infection.

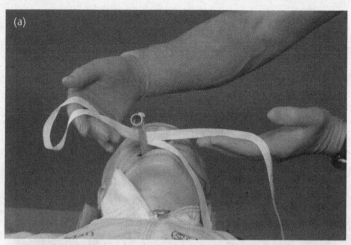

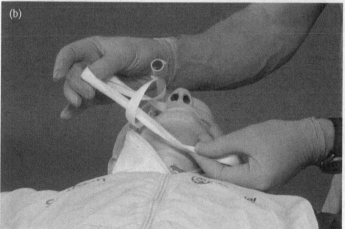

Figure 10.1 Method for securely tying the tracheal tube in position:
(a) A loop of ribbon is made above the tracheal tube: the two free ends should be of different lengths so the final knot is located away from the midline.
(b) Both ends of the ribbon are passed through the loop, forming a 'slip knot' around the tracheal tube: this automatically tightens as tension is applied.

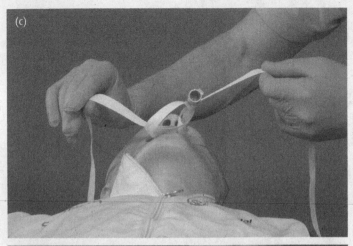

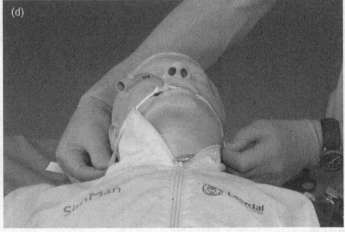

Figure 10.1 (*cont.*)
(c) The two ends of ribbon are separated, and the loop is pulled tight around the tube.
(d) The two ends of the ribbon are passed in opposite directions around the patient's neck, and secured away from the midline with an appropriate knot.

Breathing

Is ventilation satisfactory?

This is initially assessed clinically, based on chest expansion and breath sounds, but is augmented by pulse oximetry, E_TCO_2 measurement and arterial blood gas analyses.

Initially, the patient's lungs are ventilated manually, which enables an assessment of chest compliance and assists in the detection of any respiratory obstruction. If possible, the patient's lungs are then ventilated with a portable ventilator: this gives constant ventilatory support and helps achieve a steady state. Check arterial blood gases when mechanical ventilation is commenced and 20 minutes later to guide adjustment of ventilator settings.

Patients with very stiff lungs, such as those with pulmonary oedema, or with a prolonged expiratory phase, such as those with severe asthma, may need hand ventilation until a ventilator of higher specification is available.

Ventilator settings will depend initially on clinical assessment of chest expansion. A brief guide to the features of a transport ventilator is given below. Use the manufacturer's instructions and your medical physics or anaesthetic technical services department to instruct you on your particular ventilator.

The tidal volumes delivered by a ventilator may be volume controlled or pressure controlled. Transport ventilators are most commonly used in a volume-control mode as this is simpler to set up and delivers a reliable minute ventilation. Set the ventilator to deliver a tidal volume of 6–8 mL kg^{-1} ideal body weight. This will be approximately 400–500 mL for a 60–70 kg woman and 500–600 mL for a 70–80 kg man. Adjust the rate to achieve an acceptable E_TCO_2, guided primarily by the pH. Set the peak pressure limit alarm to 40 cmH$_2$O, although it is preferable to limit inspiratory pressure to 30 cmH$_2$O. This will enable most patients to be ventilated safely. In some modes of ventilation the ventilator does not interact with a patient's efforts to breathe, while in others (e.g. synchronized intermittent mandatory ventilation (SIMV)) it detects and interacts with those efforts. Continuous mandatory ventilation (CMV) is the most commonly used non-interactive volume-control mode in the emergency setting. SIMV enables the patient to initiate ventilator breaths. This is useful if neuromuscular blocking drugs have not been given, if the patient has recovered from neuromuscular blockade, or if weaning or assessing the presence of respiratory effort. Where a patient does not initiate breaths, the set SIMV breath rate is delivered in the same way as CMV (giving a backup minute volume). Regular suction of secretions is also important.

Transport ventilators (Figures 10.2, 10.3 and 10.4)

All transport ventilators have a CMV mode. Some also have SIMV, and can deliver CPAP, and others also have a pressure control ventilation mode.

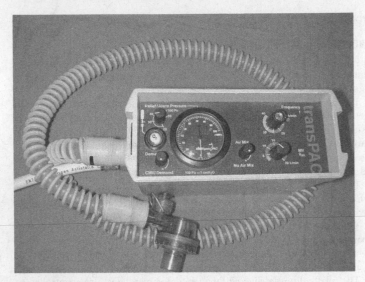

Figure 10.2 Pneupac TransPAC transport ventilator.

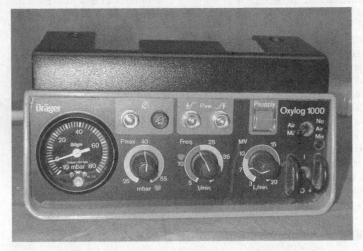

Figure 10.3 Dräger Oxylog 1000 transport ventilator.

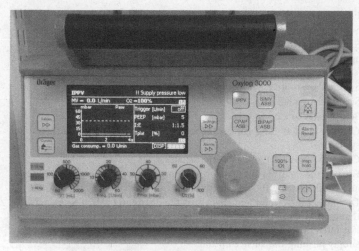

Figure 10.4 Dräger Oxylog 3000 transport ventilator.

Some less sophisticated transport ventilators deliver a set minute volume (MV) that is divided into a number of breaths per minute (respiratory rate – RR). A disadvantage of this is that decreasing the RR without altering MV will increase the tidal volume (V_T) and ventilation pressures. A peak airway pressure limiting (P_{max}) valve must be incorporated to protect against this. Later models have controls for V_T and RR to overcome this problem as well as pressure limiting valves and alarms. A disconnect alarm should be standard, but is not present on all transport ventilators: models without an integral disconnection alarm must be monitored very carefully because they will continue to cycle even if there is no patient attached. Simpler models have a fixed inspiratory:expiratory (I:E) ratio of 1:2. Others enable selection of I:E ratios over a wider range. F_iO_2 is normally 100% or 60% (air mix) on basic models or can be varied more widely on other models.

Use of positive end expiratory pressure (PEEP) is recommended in most patients. This will improve oxygenation and decrease the F_iO_2 required, primarily through recruitment of alveoli. In the hypotensive patient, use of high PEEP values will increase intrathoracic pressure and reduce venous return to the heart, which may exacerbate the hypotension. If a simple transport ventilator does not have this capacity, a PEEP valve can be attached at the patient end of the circuit.

Initial ventilator set up using the Oxylog 3000 as an example

Before attaching to the patient perform a quick ventilator check:

- Connect O_2 supply via a Schraeder valve to the wall supply or cylinder and turn the ventilator on. It will perform its own self-test which can be aborted.

- For a 'standard' adult set F_iO_2 to 1.0 by selecting 100% oxygen.
- Set the mode to intermittent positive pressure ventilation (IPPV).
- Set a V_T of 6 to 8 mL kg^{-1} (500 mL for a 'standard' adult) and an appropriate RR to achieve a MV of 100 mL kg^{-1} (15 breaths/minute for a 'standard' adult).
- Set the P_{max} to 40 cmH$_2$O.
- Set PEEP to 5 cmH$_2$O.
- Set I:E ratio to 1:2.
- Connect to a test 'lung' (or use the reservoir bag of an anaesthetic breathing system).
- Check that the 'lung' inflates and deflates.
- Squeeze the 'lung' to simulate obstruction or increasing airway pressures and check that the P_{max} alarm sounds.
- Disconnect the circuit and check that the disconnect alarm sounds. Note that the alarm can be silenced for 25 seconds by pressing the silence button; it is often preferable to silence an alarm by correcting the fault, rather than simply pushing the silence button.
- Connect to the patient. Adjust V_T according to clinical chest expansion and peak airway pressures (< 20 cmH$_2$O with normal lungs).

Ventilator trouble shooting

It is safest to switch to hand ventilation whilst solving a ventilation problem and work from the patient first, then back to the ventilator.

Consider the causes of ventilation failure:

P – position of tube (oesophageal or bronchial intubation, tube out of trachea);

O – obstruction (tubing obstruction, tracheal/bronchial obstruction or broncho-constriction e.g. severe asthma);

P – pneumothorax (particularly tension pneumothorax) or pleural effusion;

E – equipment (incorrect kit or connections/equipment failure/inadequate gas flow);

S – splinting (abdominal distension including stomach distension or poor paralysis).

A good starting point when assessing a ventilation problem is to hand-ventilate the patient. If the problem persists, then there is a patient-related problem. If you can adequately hand ventilate the patient then systematically check for ventilator or circuit issues. A check list is shown in Table 10.1.

Table 10.1 Ventilator trouble shooting

Problem	Solution
Not ventilating: no noise or pressure	Check on/off (I/O) switch Check O_2 source/connections
Not ventilating: noise but no pressure generated	Check for disconnections Check ventilation valve Check for tracheal cuff leak
Not ventilating: noise and pressure generated (high pressure)	Check for tubing kinks or obstruction (Patient may have been fighting the ventilator, may have stiff lungs or a tension pneumothorax)
Hypoxaemia	Check clinical air entry Increase F_iO_2 Increase PEEP Consider tracheal suction
Hypercapnoea Hypocapnoea	Increase MV by increasing RR Decrease MV by decreasing RR

Are tube positions correct?

Obtain a chest radiograph to check the position of the tracheal and nasogastric tubes.

Has a nasogastric or orogastric tube been placed?

Insertion of a tube into the stomach enables deflation of a dilated stomach and removal of stomach contents. This helps to reduce the potential for aspiration and may sometimes enable lower ventilation pressures. It also enables diagnosis of haemorrhage and provides access to the GI tract for drug administration.

Are chest drains required?

Chest trauma, particularly rib fractures, is associated with pneumothoraces. Small pneumothoraces may not be visible on chest radiograph, especially if they are anterior, and a tension pneumothorax may develop from a simple pneumothorax. This is a particular risk when positive pressure ventilation is commenced. Prophylactic chest drains may be inserted, particularly if the patient is about to be transported or undergo a lengthy procedure when the chest will not be immediately accessible. This is not a procedure without risk, and should be performed with care only by a suitably trained practitioner.

If a chest drain is not inserted then careful monitoring is essential, with rapid intervention to drain the chest if there is any evidence of a developing pneumothorax. Secure chest drains carefully before transfer.

Circulation

Decisions about the use of fluids and inotropes will depend on the diagnosis. Clinical assessment, which includes capillary refill time and urine output, is most important. An arterial line is considered standard if the patient is haemodynamically unstable or at risk of becoming unstable. Non-invasive BP measurement is less reliable during transfer and drains monitor batteries. A central venous catheter may be useful in securing venous access and to enable administration of inotropes. It is not a reliable guide of volume status.

In most cases, it is appropriate to maintain a mean arterial pressure of 70 mmHg or more. Exceptions to this include:

- Penetrating injury or uncontrolled haemorrhage, when hypotensive resuscitation may be appropriate.
- Head injury when it is recommended that a higher mean arterial pressure (typically 90 mmHg) is required to maintain an adequate cerebral perfusion pressure.

Hypotension

Hypotension occurs commonly after rapid sequence induction.

- Exclude hypovolaemia.
- All anaesthetic drugs can cause hypotension – adequate intravascular volume is required before and after induction. If induction causes hypotension, fluid boluses and vasopressor drugs (such as adrenaline or metaraminol) may be required.
- Exclude tension pneumothorax. Suspect and examine for this if airway pressures are increased, especially in trauma. Needle decompression or thoracostomy followed by chest drain insertion are required.
- Excessive PEEP may cause hypotension by reducing venous return, particularly if there is pre-existing myocardial impairment or hypovolaemia.
- Hyperventilation with air trapping, often in the context of obstructive airways disease, can reduce venous return and increase the risk of pneumothorax. A period of disconnection of the breathing system from the tracheal tube will enable adequate time for exhalation of trapped alveolar gas. Continue ventilation with a reduced rate and longer expiratory time. Use bronchodilators to relieve bronchospasm. A fluid challenge of 500–1000 mL will often help to restore adequate pre-load.
- Hypotension in the presence of septic shock will require treatment with a vasopressor. Noradrenaline is the first choice vasopressor in the current surviving sepsis guidelines.

- Record a 12-lead ECG to help assess causes for cardiogenic shock.
- Bedside ultrasound can be used to help assess for haemorrhage, left ventricular filling, pneumothorax and cardiac function.

Hypertension

Usually indicates inadequate analgesia or sedation unless associated with severe head injury, or raised intracranial pressure from other causes.

Disability

Check the adequacy of:

- sedation;
- analgesia;
- neuromuscular blockade;
- seizure control.

Sedation and analgesia

Consider sedation before undertaking an RSI and tracheal intubation so that post-intubation awareness is avoided and ventilation is made easier. If there is time, prepare a sedation infusion before the start of an RSI. Sedation techniques vary; usually, a sedative drug is combined with an opioid. Propofol infusions are convenient and are used widely. Anticonvulsant properties make it suitable for head injury or status epilepticus; it is also a bronchodilator and therefore useful for patients with asthma. Use propofol with care in patients with hypovolaemia. The concurrent use of opioids reduces the dose of propofol required to maintain adequate sedation. Propofol infusions are not used in children because of a propensity to cause metabolic acidosis and cardiac dysfunction (propofol infusion syndrome).

Midazolam is an alternative sedative drug. It has more cardiovascular stability, and is often combined with morphine or fentanyl. The advantage of these drugs is that they can be given by bolus, which may be useful during transport. Remifentanil, an ultra short-acting opioid, is used increasingly in intensive care units but is relatively expensive.

Neuromuscular blocking drugs

In many situations it is appropriate to paralyze intubated patients. This is particularly important for transfers. The risk of extubation is reduced, ventilation is facilitated, and sudden increases in intracranial pressure caused by gagging are avoided.

Seizure control

Seizures are controlled in the normal way with benzodiazepines such as lorazepam or diazepam. Propofol or midazolam are also effective anticonvulsants. It is common practice to give a loading dose of phenytoin or levetiracetam after a second seizure.

Exposure and environment

The exposure required for the secondary survey, combined with the vasodilatory effects of anaesthetic drugs, may cause significant cooling. This is generally harmful except, possibly, in those who have been resuscitated from cardiac arrest, and possibly some patients with head injuries.

Temperature should be monitored and warming blankets used where appropriate; warmed fluids and warmed humidified oxygen are also effective.

Transfer to definitive management

Intubated patients in the emergency department will usually require transfer from the resuscitation room to another department in the hospital, or to another hospital for continuing care. It is not always possible for the patient to be physiologically stable before transfer. For example, the patient may require transfer directly to the operating room for laparotomy after completion of the primary survey. However, the patient should be as stable as possible before transfer. Common destinations include the CT scanner, operating room and ICU in the same hospital, and specialist centres such as neurosurgery in other hospitals.

During transfer the patient is at significant risk of adverse events, and these are associated with a worse outcome. Many of these adverse events are avoidable if attention is paid to the preparation of the patient before transfer.

Always consider the worst-case scenario and, as a general rule, if you have considered an intervention before transfer (e.g. chest drains) then it probably needs doing before you leave.

A checklist for transfer appears in Box 10.1.

Preparation

Preparation follows the system described in previous sections of this chapter.

Personnel

An appropriately trained person who is aware of the risks of transportation must attend an intubated patient at all times. They should have specific training in the transportation of the critically ill. Ideally, a specialist retrieval team should transport children as this reduces critical incidents.

Box 10.1 Checklist for transfer

- Airway safe. Tube position confirmed by end tidal CO_2 monitoring and chest X-ray.
- Patient paralyzed, sedated and ventilated.
- Adequate gas exchange confirmed by ABG.
- Naso/orogastric tube in place.
- Chest tubes secured, where applicable. (Heimlich valve preferred to underwater seal).
- Circulation stable, haemorrhage controlled.
- Abdominal injuries properly assessed and treated.
- Minimum of two routes of venous access – well secured.
- Adequate haemoglobin concentration.
- Seizures controlled.
- Long bone and pelvic fractures stabilized.
- Temperature maintained.
- Acid–base, glucose and metabolic abnormalities corrected.
- Case notes, X-rays and transfer documentation.
- Cross-matched blood products with the patient, if appropriate.
- Appropriate equipment and drugs. All devices compatible with ambulance equipment. Spare batteries. Sufficient oxygen supplies for the journey (see below).
- Communication with receiving clinicians and relatives.

Accompanying staff transferring patients between hospitals should have high visibility protective and warm clothing and a means of communicating with the hospital, i.e. a mobile phone. They should be insured for injury and have an identified method of returning to their base hospital.

Equipment

All equipment used during transport should be reliable, portable and robust. Accompanying staff should be familiar with the equipment. Battery life should be long enough for transfer or an alternative should be easily available, such as an adapter to connect to the ambulance power source. Oxygen requirements need to be calculated. The recommended formula is described in Box 10.2.

During transport, ensure equipment is secured and not lying free on the patient or on the floor of the ambulance. An equipment bridge mounted over the patient and attached to the transport trolley, or a specially designed transport trolley, is ideal. These must be compatible with local ambulance service equipment. Physiological parameters, including heart rate, invasive blood pressure, oxygen saturation and quantitative end tidal CO_2, should be

Box 10.2 Calculating the oxygen required for patient transfer

Oxygen calculation:
2 × transport time in minutes × [(MV × F_iO_2) + ventilator driving gas (if appropriate)].
Give yourself at least one hour of extra O_2.
F_iO_2 is a proportion of 1, e.g. 60% = 0.6.
Ventilator driving gas varies, but is commonly 1 L min⁻¹, e.g. for MV of 10 L min⁻¹ at an F_iO_2 of 0.6 over a 1 hour trip:
O_2 required = 2 × 60 × [(10 × 0.6) + 1] = 840 L = 2 size E or 1 size F oxygen cylinder.
Note: 1 size E cylinder (680 L) at 15 L min⁻¹ flow will last only 45 minutes. There are newer high-pressure cylinders: e.g. the size HX cylinder contains 2300 L.

visible to the clinician at all times on a multiple parameter transport monitor. The ability to measure central venous pressures and core temperature should also be available. A transport bag or rucksack containing emergency drugs, fluids and airway equipment should be carried during transfer.

Documentation

Review and update the clinical records. Record observations regularly, usually at 15-minute intervals. The standard of observation should be the same as in an ICU throughout the assessment and resuscitation period, and during transfer. Organize outstanding investigations and review and document results. Complete a pre-transfer checklist before transfer. Ensure that all relevant documentation, including drug charts, fluid charts and copies of investigations such as x-rays go with the patient. In some cases cross-matched blood will also be required.

Communication

There should be clear communication between all clinical specialties involved in the patient's care. If referral or care is discussed via the telephone, document this communication clearly in the clinical records. This should include the names of the clinicians and the time and date. Ensure that the receiving department is aware of the departure of the patient from the resuscitation room; for example, the CT scanner is free and available *before* the patient leaves the emergency department. A receiving hospital should also receive adequate warning of the patient's arrival. If the accompanying staff have not been involved in the patient's care before transfer, adequate handover must take place before transportation. Speak to the patient's relatives before transfer to definitive care. Give them directions to the receiving hospital department and inform them whom they should speak to. There should be a recognized method for contacting the local ambulance service and ensuring rapid availability of a fully equipped ambulance for transfer. Ambulance personnel must know the location of the receiving hospital and department before transfer. Discuss with ambulance personnel the urgency of the transfer and requirement for blue lights.

Considerations during transport

The patient is most at risk when they are being moved; for example, transfer into the CT scanner or from the resuscitation room to the ambulance. At this time there is a significant possibility that the tracheal tube or intravascular access will become dislodged. Careful coordination and attention to detail during these manoeuvres will reduce the likelihood of these events happening. Handover and transfer to the bed at the receiving department is also a time of risk and the patient should be settled and all monitoring, drug infusions and ventilation transferred and continued before formal handover occurs.

If preparation has been thorough, there should be little to do during transport, apart from continuous monitoring of the patient. Ensure that monitors are clearly visible and intravascular access secured and accessible at all times. Prepare drugs that may be required during transfer before departure; label them and ensure that they are immediately accessible to the accompanying staff. The aim is for no intervention to be necessary during transport. If the patient requires attention during transfer, consider stopping the ambulance. Document and review any critical incidents that occur.

Extubation

It may occasionally be appropriate to extubate a patient in the emergency department; for example, after a scan or on recovery after a cardiac arrest. This decision is made only by a senior physician and only when extubation criteria have been met. There should be full motor power and no residual neuromuscular blockade. Estimate the likely duration of action of the muscle relaxant and the need for reversal with neostigmine and glycopyrrolate; if necessary, give neostigmine 50 mcg kg^{-1} and glycopyrrolate 10 mcg kg^{-1} and wait 10–15 minutes for the reversal to be fully effective. If rocuronium has been used, consider using sugammadex, but this is an expensive option.

The adequacy of reversal is usually assessed clinically, determining muscle power by asking the patient to maintain head lift for 5 seconds. If the patient appears to be twitching at eye opening they may be inadequately reversed; continue the sedation and assess again in 15–20 minutes.

The patient must have adequate cardiorespiratory function to maintain oxygenation without the aid of the ventilator. As a rule of thumb, if the patient does not have a P_aO_2 greater than 10 kPa on 40% inspired oxygen concentration, or an S_pO_2 greater than 95%, then they are unlikely to oxygenate adequately once extubated. They should also be able to generate tidal volumes of at least 500 mL through the anaesthetic breathing system without any inspiratory support and the respiratory rate should be less than 20 breaths per minute.

If all these criteria are met, the patient may be extubated. Ensure the oropharynx is adequately clear of secretions by suction, sit the patient up and have appropriate oxygen delivery systems ready. Suction the trachea, deflate the cuff and remove the tube. Ensure that reintubation can be achieved quickly if required.

Summary

- The post-intubation phase is an integral part of emergency airway management.
- The objectives of the post-intubation phase are to achieve sufficient physiological stability for transfer and to carry out other appropriate treatment.
- A modified ABCDE system provides useful prompts to correct and complete patient management.
- Practitioners must be familiar with the drugs and equipment commonly used in the post-intubation phase.
- Thorough and systematic preparation is essential for safe patient transfer.
- Extubation may be indicated early in some patients following emergency RSI, and can be achieved safely if certain conditions are met.

Acknowledgement

This chapter has been updated from the first edition chapter, which was written by Paul Younge, David Lockey and Alasdair Gray.

Further reading

1   Association of Anaesthetists of Great Britain and Ireland. (2007) Standards of Monitoring During Anaesthesia and Recovery (4th edition). London: Association of Anaesthetists of Great Britain and Ireland. Available at: http://www.aagbi.org/sites/default/files/standardsofmonitoring07.pdf (accessed November 2014).

2   Intensive Care Society. (2011) Standards and Guidelines: Transport of the Critically Ill Adult (3rd edition). London: Intensive Care Society. Available at: http://www.ics.ac.uk/ics-homepage/guidelines-standards/ (accessed November 2014).

3   Association of Anaesthetists of Great Britain and Ireland. (2006) Recommendations for the safe transfer of patients with brain injury. London: Association of Anaesthetists of Great Britain and Ireland. Available at: http://www.aagbi.org/sites/default/files/braininjury.pdf (accessed November 2014).

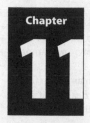

Chapter 11

Emergency airway management in special circumstances

11.1 Paediatrics

Patricia Weir and Paul Younge

Objectives

The objectives of this section are to:

- Understand the principles of emergency airway management that apply to children.
- Understand the key airway differences between adults and children.
- Appreciate the need to obtain early specialist help with paediatric airway management.

Introduction

The need to intubate children using drugs outside an operating room is rare. Even in busy centres this will occur only around once a month. It is therefore difficult to obtain and maintain the necessary skills. In most institutions skilled airway assistance in the form of an experienced anaesthetist will be available quickly and their help should always be sought.

> Do not attempt RSI in children unless:
> a. you have appropriate skills and training, or;
> b. in an emergency – the patient's airway, and adequate oxygenation, cannot be maintained using basic airway manoeuvres such as an oropharyngeal airway and bag-mask ventilation, and assistance is *not imminent*.

Emergency Airway Management, Second Edition, ed. Andrew Burtenshaw, Jonathan Benger and Jerry Nolan. Published by Cambridge University Press. © College of Emergency Medicine, London, 2015.

Special considerations in children

1. Anatomical: (Figure 11.1)
   - Head size (large occiput) – causes neck flexion.
   - The infant's tongue is relatively large in proportion to the rest of the oral cavity. It therefore more easily obstructs the airway, and is more difficult to manipulate with a laryngoscope blade.
   - The infant's larynx is higher in the neck (C3-4) than in an adult (C4-5).
   - The epiglottis is angled away from the axis of the trachea, and it is therefore more difficult to lift the epiglottis with the tip of a laryngoscope blade.
   - The narrowest portion of the infant larynx is the cricoid cartilage (compared to the vocal cords in an adult). Therefore a tracheal tube will pass through the cords and be tightly wedged against the tracheal wall at the level of the cricoid, causing damage to the tracheal mucosa and potential subglottic stenosis or post-extubation stridor.
   - The trachea is relatively short, increasing the risk of bronchial intubation or extubation during patient transfer.
   - No teeth in infancy.

   The child develops adult anatomy by the age of 10–12 years. The greatest anatomical differences exist in the infant (i.e. < 1 year).

2. Physiological:
   - High basal oxygen consumption (6 mL kg^{-1} min^{-1}, or twice that of adults).

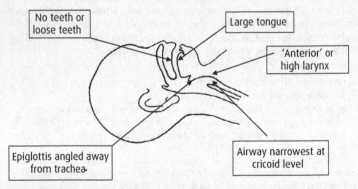

No teeth or loose teeth

Large tongue

'Anterior' or high larynx

Epiglottis angled away from trachea

Airway narrowest at cricoid level

Figure 11.1 Anatomical features of a child's airway that differ from an adult.

- Lower functional residual capacity (FRC).
- Children therefore have significantly less oxygen reserve and will desaturate much faster than adults.

3. Weight:

If the child's weight is not known the following formulae can be used:

0–12 months weight in kg = (0.5 × age in months) + 4
1–5 years   weight in kg = (2 × age in years) + 8
6–12 years   weight in kg = (3 × age in years) + 7

4. Drugs:

- Drug dosage. The effective doses of induction drugs such as propofol and thiopental sodium are relatively greater in children of 6 months to 16 years (Table 11.1).

Ensure an adequate dose of suxamethonium! Remember to have a follow-up dose of a non-depolarizing neuromuscular blocker drawn up to give once the airway is secure (e.g. rocuronium 1 mg kg^{-1}, vecuronium 0.1 mg kg^{-1}, atracurium 0.6 mg kg^{-1}).

- Pre-treatment with anticholinergics is not undertaken routinely. However, always give atropine 0.02 mg kg^{-1} before a second dose of suxamethonium and ensure that the correct dose of atropine is drawn up and ready to give before RSI is undertaken in children.

5. Cricoid pressure:

The application of cricoid pressure in neonates and young infants (< 6 months) is controversial. If applied poorly, it may distort the larynx resulting in a poor or no view of the vocal cords. Therefore, some clinicians advocate not applying it in this age group. If cricoid pressure is

Table 11.1 Drug doses for induction and neuromuscular blockade in children

Induction	Stable child	Propofol 2.5–3 mg kg^{-1}, or, thiopental sodium 3–5 mg kg^{-1}
	Unstable child	Ketamine 2 mg kg^{-1} and fentanyl 1–2 mcg kg^{-1}, or midazolam 0.05–0.1 mg kg^{-1}
Neuromuscular blockers	Weight < 20 kg	Suxamethonium* 2 mg kg^{-1} flushed with normal saline
	Weight > 20 kg	Suxamethonium 1–2 mg kg^{-1}

* Fasciculation is not seen in young children

Table 11.2 Optimal patient positioning for effective airway management in children of various ages

Preterm/ex-prem	Neutral position – may require a small roll under shoulders to compensate for large occiput.
Infant (up to 1 year)	Neutral position – because of the large occiput naturally resulting in neck flexion.
Small child (< 8 years)	Head tilt, chin lift resulting in neck flexion/head extension.
Older child (> 8 years)	With increasing age a small pillow may need to be placed under the child's head to achieve optimal conditions.

applied and the larynx is not seen then the practitioner should either ask the assistant to let go, or should undertake bimanual laryngoscopy, using external laryngeal manipulation to improve the view.

6. Position:

Positioning is age dependent because of the anatomical considerations outlined above. The optimal position for intubation is the same as for bag-mask ventilation (Table 11.2).

There is a tendency for the infant head to roll from side to side; this can be controlled by the use of a sandbag, fluid bag or towel at the side of the head.

Equipment

Oropharyngeal airways

These are available from size 000 (absolutely tiny and rarely required) to adult size.

Sizing of oropharyngeal airways is important because an airway that is too small will get buried in the tongue and one too large may hit and push down the epiglottis (Figures 11.2 and 11.3). Measurement from the incisor teeth to the angle of the jaw will give approximately the correct size. If the child appears to be swallowing the airway, it is too small, and if it fails to seat fully in the mouth, it is too big. The technique for insertion in children is the same as for adults, but rough manipulation will cause trauma. In infants the airway should be inserted the correct way up (i.e. the way that it will ultimately sit), using a laryngoscope blade or a tongue depressor to facilitate placement.

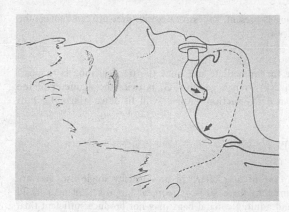

Figure 11.2
Position of an
oropharyngeal
airway that is
too short.

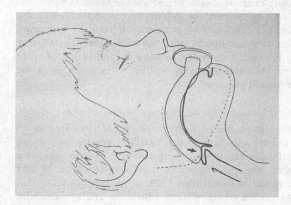

Figure 11.3
Position of an
oropharyngeal
airway that is
too long.

Facemasks

Clear plastic cuffed facemasks enable good contour fit onto the face, and detection of colour change, vomit or misting of the mask.

Suction

Yankauer

Must be available, connected and functioning at induction. These come in a variety of sizes and with or without an aperture in the shaft. Covering the aperture with a finger allows fine control of the suction. It is important to be aware if an aperture is present. Excessive negative pressure can damage the soft tissues of the airway.

Narrow-bore

Should be available for immediate use once the tracheal tube is in position. The correct size in French gauge (FG) is twice the diameter of the tracheal tube (i.e. an 8 FG suction catheter will fit down a size 4.0 mm tracheal tube).

Breathing systems
Self-inflating bags

These are safe and easy to use. They are now usually single use, and are generally manufactured in three sizes – neonatal (approx. 250 mL), child (approx. 500 mL) and adult. Neonatal bags may not produce sufficient tidal volumes when used in non-neonates, especially if there is a poor seal around the facemask. Therefore their use should be restricted to neonates only.

Some self-inflating bags designed for children have a pressure relief valve set at around 45 cmH$_2$O. This can be overridden if required by placing a finger on the valve. It is not usually necessary to do this; however, if it is deemed necessary to override the valve, consider the potentially reversible causes of high airway resistance such as obstruction or blockage in the breathing system or tension pneumothorax.

Ayres T-piece

(Mapleson F breathing system, Jackson Rees modification of Ayres T-piece)

It is important to have specific paediatric breathing systems for younger children. The Ayres T-piece requires some experience and a fresh gas source to use, but is popular with anaesthetists as it enables assessment of lung compliance and the ability to switch from IPPV to spontaneous ventilation with ease. These systems are generally single patient use and available with 500 mL or 1 litre bags.

Sufficient fresh gas flow (FGF) is required when using an Ayres T-piece to minimize rebreathing of expired CO$_2$.

For spontaneous ventilation: FGF = $2 - 3 \times$ minute ventilation
For IPPV: FGF = $1000\,\text{mL} + 200\,\text{mL}\,\text{kg}^{-1}$

Laryngoscopes

Differences in the anatomy of the larynx in infants (i.e. < 1 year) make a straight-bladed laryngoscope the instrument of choice in this age group. This is placed beneath the epiglottis and lifted to expose the larynx.

Straight-bladed laryngoscopes are narrower and preferred by many anaesthetists for children under five years, as they allow more room in the mouth; alternatively, a size 2 Macintosh (curved blade) can be used in this age group. Disposable blades, which are slightly thicker, generally have a very good light and are now in common use. It is advisable to have alternative blades available.

Videolaryngoscopy is used increasingly in paediatric practice and for training purposes.

Tracheal tubes

A non-cuffed tracheal tube (TT) is classically used in the pre-pubertal child to minimize damage to the tracheal mucosa. The correct size in children over one year can be calculated using the following formulae:

Non-cuffed TT sizing
Internal diameter = (age in years/4) + 4

Cuffed TT sizing
Cuff should be inflated; therefore a smaller diameter is required. Commonly one size smaller than predicted by the formula above (e.g. 3.0 rather than 3.5) (see manufacturers instructions)

The 0.5 mm size above and below should always be available. Term babies will generally require a 3.5 mm tracheal tube.

In elective surgery, it was traditionally optimal to have a slight leak of air around the tracheal tube when applying 20 cmH_2O pressure: this ensures that the tube is not tightly wedged against the tracheal mucosa. However, in an emergency, there is often decreased lung compliance and it is usually desirable to have no or minimal leak. Cuffed TTs are now often the tube of choice in an emergency. This practice appears to be safe and has the advantage of being able to predictably achieve a correct fitting TT when lung compliance is decreased. Specifically designed paediatric cuffed TTs are available from size 2.5–3.0 upwards, depending on the manufacturer.

Smaller-sized tracheal tubes allow cuff inflation and avoid pressure points from wrinkled cuffs. Monitor cuff pressures carefully.

There is no consensus on whether or not a tracheal tube should be cut. In an emergency it is better to have a longer tracheal tube, which can be repositioned if required, than a tracheal tube that subsequently proves to be too short and may become dislodged from the trachea.

Stylets and bougies

Stylets are generally stiff wire covered in plastic, designed to stiffen the tracheal tube and enable it to be angled towards the larynx. They have the potential to cause significant trauma, and must not protrude from the distal end of the tracheal tube. Stylets are particularly useful when inserting small tracheal tubes (4.0 mm or less), which lack intrinsic rigidity. Inexperienced practitioners may find it easier to routinely mount a stylet in smaller tracheal tubes before commencing intubation.

Bougies are designed for use in difficult intubations: they are inserted into the trachea enabling a tracheal tube to be railroaded into position. Orange/red paediatric bougies are available in several sizes.

Before use, check that the tracheal tube fits over the chosen bougie and that it is well lubricated.

RSI technique in children

Checklists for intubation have been widely adopted for use in children.

Pre-oxygenation

Children must be pre-oxygenated as well as possible because their oxygen reserve is less and their arterial blood will desaturate quickly (Figure 2.11). The ideal is at least 3 minutes breathing 100% oxygen. However, this can be difficult to achieve in an uncooperative child. Before elective anaesthesia, pre-oxygenation can be achieved by encouraging the child to take 3–4 maximal inspiratory breaths.

Ideally, pre-oxygenation is carried out with a breathing system that can deliver 100% oxygen and has a low resistance to breathing, such as an Ayres T-piece. Pre-oxygenation with a self-inflating bag-mask in infants requires considerable effort; avoid it unless there is no other option.

Position patient appropriately for age and size (see above).

Equipment – have you got everything? (Box 11.1)

Laryngoscopy

A reproducible technique for intubating neonates and small infants is to introduce the laryngoscope from the right and move to the centre, ensuring the blade is in the midline. Move down over the tongue and epiglottis, past the larynx, then gently pull back until the larynx falls into view. Note how this differs from adult laryngoscopic technique.

In older children the tip of the laryngoscope blade can be placed in the vallecula (as for adults), lifting in the line of the handle to expose the vocal cords.

> **Box 11.1 Equipment for intubation**
>
> - Facemask.
> - Breathing system.
> - Oropharyngeal airways.
> - Yankauer suction catheter.
> - Laryngoscope.
> - Tracheal tubes.
> - Paediatric Magill's forceps.
> - Fine-bore suction catheters.
> - Nasogastric tube.
> - Tape/ties.
> - E_TCO_2 measurement.

Insert the tracheal tube and check for E_TCO_2 (using waveform capnography), chest movement, misting of the tube, leak and bilateral equal air entry on auscultation, louder over the lungs than the epigastrium.

> It is easy to insert the tracheal tube too far in small children, which usually results in passage into the right main bronchus.

Fixation of the tracheal tube

There are many ways to fix tracheal tubes, including commercial fixation devices. In children, taping is preferable to tying and a simple and effective method is to use 1 inch pink 'Elastoplast trouserlegs' (Figure 11.4).

Take the first piece and attach the uncut end to the right cheek. With a bit of stretch on the tape put the upper limb across the upper lip, then wind the lower limb securely around the tracheal tube. Take the second piece and attach it to the left cheek. Take the lower limb and place this across the lower lip, then wind the upper limb around the tracheal tube.

If the patient is going to be transported, provide additional stability by inserting an oropharyngeal airway and applying a third piece of Elastoplast with a central hole cut to accommodate the tracheal tube.

a. Have two pieces of Elastoplast tape, cut ready for use.
b. Take the first piece and attach the uncut end to the right cheek. With a bit of stretch on the tape put the upper limb across the upper lip.
c. Wind the lower limb securely around the tracheal tube.
d. Take the second piece and attach the uncut end to the left cheek.
e. Stretch the lower limb and place this across the lower lip, then wind the upper limb securely around the tracheal tube.
f. Tracheal tube taped securely in position.

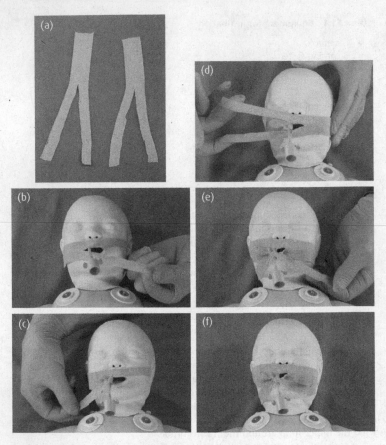

Figure 11.4 Elastoplast fixation of the tracheal tube in children.

Ventilators

Most children >10 kg can be ventilated using commonly available transport ventilators. Smaller tidal volumes (e.g. <100 mL) can be difficult to achieve with an unmodified transport ventilator; use a purpose designed paediatric transport ventilator.

The difficult airway in children

Difficult airways are uncommon in normal children, but they do occur in association with acute upper airway obstruction and craniofacial anomalies (e.g. Pierre Robin, Goldenhar's, etc.). These can usually be anticipated by observation of the child's facial features or clinical status. If a difficult airway is anticipated, seek senior anaesthetic help. Seek help early in acute upper airway obstruction or in children with syndromes that affect the airway.

The Association of Paediatric Anaesthetists has produced a series of guidelines linked to the Difficult Airway Society for management of difficult paediatric airways (see Further reading).

Summary

- There are significant differences between adults and children. Do not attempt RSI and tracheal intubation in young children unless you have appropriate training and experience. Always seek the help of an experienced paediatric anaesthetist.
- Children desaturate quickly: pre-oxygenate as thoroughly as possible.
- Check that you have *all* the correct equipment for children before commencing RSI and tracheal intubation.

Further reading

1 Advanced Life Support Group. (2005) *Advanced Paediatric Life Support. The Practical Approach*, 4th edn. London: BMJ Books/Blackwells.

2 Carwell, M., Walker, R.W.M. (2003) Management of the difficult paediatric airway. Contin Educ Anaesth Crit Care Pain; 3: 167–70.

3 Bhardwaj, N. (2013) Paediatric cuffed endotracheal tubes. J Anaesthesiol Clin Pharmacol; 29(1): 13–18.

4 APA difficult airway guidelines 2012. Available at: www.APAgbi.org.uk (accessed November 2014).

11.2 Major trauma and raised intracranial pressure

Jonathan Hulme and Dinendra S. Gill

Objectives

The objectives of this section are to:

- Understand the importance of emergency airway management in minimizing secondary brain injury.
- Recognize the importance of extracranial injuries in the resuscitation of patients with traumatic brain injury (TBI).
- Appreciate the principles of safe transfer of major trauma patients.

Introduction

Major trauma remains the commonest cause of death in the first four decades of life; however, mortality is decreasing following the creation of trauma networks in the UK. Established trauma courses emphasize the importance of a structured approach to simultaneous rapid assessment and resuscitation, and the concept of damage control resuscitation (DCR) is now applied widely in the management of trauma patients. DCR starts with management of the airway (with cervical spine control), breathing and circulation (haemorrhage control and haemostatic resuscitation with blood products). In some patients, control of external catastrophic haemorrhage will take priority over immediate airway intervention, but this is uncommon in civilian practice.

A brief conversation with the patient will provide important information about airway patency, adequacy of breathing and circulation, and a rough estimate of the Glasgow Coma Scale (GCS) score. Apply high-flow oxygen immediately via a mask with a reservoir bag. Make a rapid decision about immediate, urgent or observant management of the airway (see Chapter 5). If the patient is in the immediate or urgent categories, a plan is made for intubation, with consideration of the drugs to be used and a failed intubation strategy to be followed if there are problems achieving intubation, and adequate oxygenation and ventilation must be established.

Make an assessment of the likely difficulty of intubation and ventilation. Trauma patients have a higher rate of failed intubation due to disrupted airway anatomy (e.g. maxillofacial/neck trauma), soiled airway and the requirement for cervical spine control. Videolaryngoscopy now has an important role to play in improving first time intubation rates in these patients, although airway contamination with blood may impair videolaryngoscopic views.

Airway

In the trauma patient, the airway may be compromised by:

- secretions, vomit, blood;
- foreign bodies;
- burns, smoke inhalation;
- maxillofacial injuries;
- depressed conscious level;
- blunt or penetrating injury to the neck.

Airway management will depend on the urgency of intubation, the experience of the practitioner, the ability to get experienced help quickly and the equipment available.

Rapid sequence induction is indicated in trauma and head injury in the following circumstances:

- failure of the patient to maintain their own airway;
- inadequate spontaneous breathing;
- depressed conscious level;
- anticipated deterioration in airway, breathing or conscious level;
- anticipated clinical course, or on humanitarian grounds. (e.g. multiple injuries);
- where airway management will facilitate safe transfer.

Cervical spine management

Cervical spine injury (CSI) is assumed in all major trauma victims and patients with moderate or severe head injury. Stabilize the cervical spine with a rigid cervical collar, head blocks and tapes, or by using in-line manual stabilization. Clinical decision rules have been developed to assist in ruling out CSI, but these can be applied only to patients who are alert and cooperative. Early cervical spine clearance is impossible when the patient is obtunded, and the whole spine must be protected from uncontrolled movement until further investigations are completed.

Patients may arrive in an emergency department on a scoop stretcher, vacuum mattress or long (extrication) board. A long board is removed as soon as possible because of the risk of causing pressure sores. To minimize spinal and overall patient movement most patients may remain on a scoop stretcher or vacuum mattress for CT imaging, according to local protocols.

Orotracheal intubation following RSI is the technique of choice in head-injured patients, and those at risk of CSI. The hard collar, head blocks and tape are removed, and replaced with manual in-line stabilization provided by a designated assistant. This person stands or kneels at the side of the patient, either above or below the head, to allow the airway practitioner unimpeded access (Figure 11.5).

Cervical spine stabilization from above the head is common when intubating on a trolley in hospital, because the assistant can kneel to the left-hand side of the intubating practitioner, causing minimal obstruction. Out of hospital, where patients may be intubated lying on the ground, it is sometimes more expedient to stabilize the cervical spine from below the head. This gives the assistant a better view and causes less obstruction to the intubating practitioner. However, this technique reduces access to the neck, and it is important to ensure that full mouth opening is not prevented by holding the head too low.

Most trauma patients will not have a cervical spine injury and even those who do are very unlikely to suffer harm from small movements of the cervical spine. Airway management always takes priority over cervical spine stabilization and in a patient where initial attempts to intubate have been unsuccessful it is reasonable to adjust the head and neck position slightly, even if the patient is at risk of spinal cord injury. Record in the notes the methods used to protect the patient from further spinal injury.

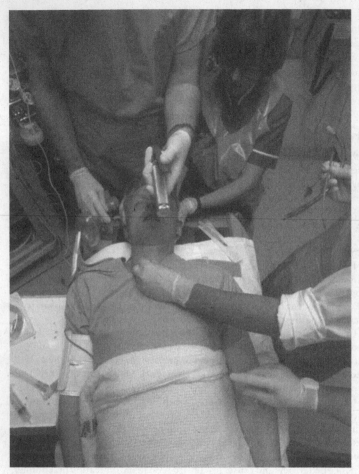

Figure 11.5 Manual in-line cervical spine stabilization during intubation.

Rapid sequence induction in trauma and traumatic brain injury

Rapid sequence induction enables optimum oxygenation and ventilation to protect the injured brain from secondary insult, and facilitates further investigation and transfer.

The technique of RSI and intubation is described in Chapters 6 and 8. A difficult airway must be anticipated in trauma, and techniques for this are described in Chapter 9.

Minimize secondary insults during RSI and intubation. Intravenous induction drugs are indicated even in obtunded patients because effective sedation and analgesia limits the increase in ICP associated with laryngoscopy and intubation. Consider pre-treatment with fentanyl or alfentanil (see Chapter 8) to reduce the sympathetic response to intubation.

There is no ideal induction drug; practitioners should choose drugs with which they are most familiar, modifying the dose according to the patient's condition.

Propofol reduces systemic vascular resistance (SVR) and will exacerbate hypotension secondary to hypovolaemia; consider using an alternative induction drug in the hypovolaemic trauma patient or the adjuvent use of a vasopressor.

Ketamine maintains blood pressure more effectively at induction, as it increases cardiac output via the sympathetic nervous system; however, in severe hypovolaemia and in patients unable to mount a sympathetic response, cardiovascular compromise may still occur at doses up to 2 mg kg^{-1}: dose reduction is recommended (e.g. 1 mg kg^{-1}).

Concerns that ketamine increases ICP significantly and is therefore contraindicated in the brain-injured patient are no longer considered valid. The priority to prevent hypotension and its associated increased mortality in patients with head injury makes ketamine a first choice for many practitioners. In the hypertensive brain-injured patient, ketamine may still remain a suitable induction drug for the same reasons; some recommend coadministration of a short-acting opiate (e.g. 1–3 mcg kg^{-1} fentanyl) to blunt the hypertensive response to laryngoscopy.

The alternative is thiopental sodium which is used in reduced doses (10–25% of normal dose), often with fentanyl, in the haemodynamically compromised patient.

Rapid onset of paralysis is achieved by high-dose rocuronium or suxamethonium depending on the practitioner's preference and experience. If using suxamethonium, give a longer-acting neuromuscular blocker (e.g. rocuronium or atracurium) when the airway is secured, to prevent coughing and straining.

> Use the drugs with which you are most familiar, but remember that considerable dose reduction may be required in critically ill and injured patients.

Breathing

Look for evidence of a tension pneumothorax, open pneumothorax or massive haemothorax and treat these immediately. Flail chest, pulmonary contusions, multiple rib fractures and simple pneumothorax all reduce the respiratory reserve. With major chest injuries, even 100% oxygen may fail to oxygenate the patient adequately and rapid desaturation is likely at induction. Optimum pre-oxygenation attempts before RSI are essential. Positive pressure ventilation can convert a simple pneumothorax into a tension pneumothorax so the presence of a pneumothorax should be diagnosed prior to intubation during the primary survey. This will be done with a combination of clinical assessment and/or radiological assessment (chest ultrasound and chest radiograph). If required, decompression of the chest with a finger thoracostomy followed by chest drain insertion should be carried out as soon as correct tracheal tube position is confirmed. Consider placing chest drains before transfer in intubated patients with small pneumothoraces and/or multiple rib fractures. If a chest drain is not placed then careful communication and monitoring is required, including a clear plan to intervene immediately if there are signs of tension pneumothorax.

Ventilator settings require adjustment in trauma patients, especially those with chest trauma who are particularly at risk of acute respiratory distress syndrome (ARDS). Excessive tidal volumes can cause ventilator associated lung injury (VALI) from overdistension of alveoli (volutrauma), repeated recruitment and collapse of alveoli (shear stress and atelectrauma), and high pressure induced damage (barotrauma). Ventilation with tidal volumes of 6–8 mL kg^{-1} ideal body weight and limitation of plateau pressure (≤ 30 cmH$_2$O) increases survival in patients with ARDS. However, hypercarbia must be avoided in TBI patients because of the risk of raised ICP; this is achieved by increasing the ventilation rate.

Circulation

All trauma patients are likely to have overt or covert blood loss. Some signs of shock, e.g. hypotension, are less likely especially in children and young adults. Tachycardia does not always occur in hypovolaemia, and cardiac pacemakers and the use of drugs such as beta-blockers also influence heart rate. It is essential that reliable vascular access is secured and that resuscitation with warmed blood products is established early via large-bore venous access. Intraosseous access is an effective alternative if intravenous access cannot be sited. Circulatory insufficiency may also have non-haemorrhagic causes such as tension pneumothorax, cardiac tamponade, myocardial contusion or neurogenic shock. Blood product resuscitation, together with the administration of tranexamic acid, is the appropriate initial treatment for circulatory shock in trauma, regardless of the underlying cause.

Hypotensive resuscitation is practiced in bleeding trauma patients until haemorrhage control is established. With the exception of patients with an isolated head injury, the target systolic blood pressure is 90 mmHg (approximately equivalent to the presence of a radial pulse). This is achieved by infusing fluid and not by giving vasopressors and/or inotropes. In the presence of hypovolaemia, vasopressors and inotropes will cause peripheral tissue hypoperfusion and may increase mortality. However, to increase cerebral perfusion in patients with isolated head injuries it is appropriate to use vasoactive drugs to maintain a higher mean arterial pressure (MAP).

Neurological injury

Traumatic brain injury is divided into primary and secondary brain injury. Primary injuries are caused by mechanical disruption to the brain occurring at the time of the initial trauma (contusion, laceration, diffuse axonal injury). Secondary injuries are subdivided into intracranial and extracranial causes (Table 11.3). Forty per cent of patients with severe TBI also have a significant extracranial injury. Hypoxaemia (SpO_2 less than 90%) and hypotension (systolic blood pressure less than 90 mmHg) increase mortality. The principal treatment aim is to prevent secondary injuries and preserve the potential for neurological recovery.

Raised ICP and reduced cerebral perfusion pressure (CPP) also increase mortality. Raised ICP is common in patients with an abnormal CT scan and persisting coma after resuscitation, and in patients over 40 years with a normal CT scan but abnormal posturing and prior episodes of arterial hypotension. In the absence of a haematoma, hypoxaemia, hypercarbia and hypotension are the commonest causes of secondary brain injury, and these insults must be anticipated and treated promptly. Early intubation is required in comatose patients with TBI and should be considered in patients with lesser degrees of impaired consciousness in association with extracranial injuries or agitation.

Table 11.3 Causes of secondary brain injury

Intracranial	Extracranial
Haematoma	Hypoxaemia
Cerebral oedema	Arterial hypotension
Seizures	Hypercarbia
Vasospasm	Hypocarbia
Infection	Anaemia
Hydrocephalus	Pyrexia
	Hyponatraemia
	Hypoglycaemia
	Hyperglycaemia

The relationship between mean arterial blood pressure (MAP), ICP and cerebral perfusion pressure (CPP) is set out below. By convention the impact of the central venous pressure (CVP), which also counters CPP, is ignored. The normal ICP is 0–10 mmHg. Traumatic brain injury patients with GCS less than 9 are likely to have an ICP of at least 20–30 mmHg. Regional hypoperfusion of the injured brain may occur when the CPP decreases below 60 mmHg. It is therefore essential to maintain a MAP of at least 90 mmHg with fluids, inotropes, vasopressors and careful selection and use of sedative and analgesic drugs. However, a MAP of 90 mmHg may be too high for polytrauma victims with ongoing haemorrhage: every effort should be made to control the haemorrhage and minimize secondary brain injury.

$$CPP = MAP - ICP$$

Post-intubation management

Once the patient has been intubated, mechanical ventilation is instituted. Sedation, with or without paralysis, relieves distress and enables effective control of oxygenation and ventilation. The ventilator is set to ensure that oxygen saturation remains above 98% and P_aO_2 greater than 12 kPa. Hyperventilation may reduce cerebral perfusion, and P_aCO_2 should not be reduced below 4.5 kPa. Avoid high positive end expiratory pressure (PEEP) and maximum inspiratory pressure (P_{max}) because these will reduce venous return from the head, causing venous congestion of the brain.

A continuous infusion of an intravenous anaesthetic and an opioid are used to maintain sedation and analgesia. The commonest combinations are propofol and fentanyl or alfentanil, or midazolam and morphine. Propofol and fentanyl/alfentanil are shorter acting and enable faster recovery of consciousness when discontinued. The use of propofol for maintenance of anaesthesia is more appropriate for patients who are haemodynamically stable. Midazolam and fentanyl can be given by bolus and may be preferred during transport, particularly in unstable patients.

Routine use of neuromuscular blockade varies between centres. If the patient is to remain paralyzed for some time, an IV infusion of a neuromuscular blocker such as atracurium can be used. Intermittent boluses of neuromuscular blocker are discouraged because delay in giving the next bolus may lead to coughing or gagging on the tracheal tube, and an increase in ICP. Long-term use of neuromuscular blockers, especially the aminosteroids (such as rocuronium and vecuronium), is associated with the development of critical care neuromyopathy.

Transport and monitoring

In patients intubated for trauma and TBI the minimum monitoring requirements are:

- ECG
- SpO_2
- E_TCO_2, with frequent validation against arterial blood gases
- Intra-arterial pressure monitoring
- Central venous pressure
- Tympanic or other form of central temperature measurement. This should be recorded frequently: disordered thermo-regulation is relatively common.

The level of sedation, muscle relaxation, GCS, pupil size and pupil reactivity are recorded at least every 15 minutes. Strict fluid balance charts are maintained, with euvolaemia the target. Insert orogastric and urinary catheters in all patients.

The principles of safe preparation for transfer are described in Chapter 10. These should be followed closely, whether the patient is transferred within the hospital (CT scan, angiography suite, operating room, intensive care unit) or to a specialist unit in another hospital. Deterioration in physiological status is common during transportation, and this has an adverse effect on outcome.

The agitated patient

Agitation after trauma may have one or more causes including hypoxaemia, shock, head injury, intoxication, pain and anxiety. Agitation must be controlled so that the patient can be properly assessed and managed without causing further injury to themselves or others. Always assume that the patient has a potentially life-threatening condition, and not that they are merely intoxicated. Sedation may be achieved using intravenous ketamine or midazolam, but only to facilitate the process of RSI. Use small, incremental doses and allow time for the drug to act before administering further doses. In some cases RSI may be performed to facilitate subsequent CT scanning, and it may be appropriate to wake the patient after the scan, and when any other urgent investigations and procedures have been completed.

Summary

- Adequate resuscitation, with avoidance of hypoxaemia, hypercarbia and arterial hypotension, improves outcome in major trauma and TBI.
- Rapid sequence induction is the technique of choice for securing the airway; it is essential to have a clear plan for failed intubation.
- All patients with major trauma have reduced physiological reserve: careful selection of drugs and dosages is required.

Acknowledgement

This chapter has been updated from the first edition chapter, which was written by Andy Eynon and Patrick Nee.

Further reading

1 Association of Anaesthetists of Great Britain and Ireland. (2006) Recommendations for the Safe Transfer of Patients with Brain Injury. London: Association of Anaesthetists of Great Britain and Ireland.

2 Jansen, J.O., Thomas, R., Loudon, M.A. *et al.* (2009) Damage control resuscitation for patients with major trauma. Brit Med J; 338: 1436–40.

3 Sperry, J.L., Minei, J.P., Frankel, H.L. *et al.* (2008) Early use of vasopressors after injury: caution before constriction. J Trauma Inj Infect Crit Care; 64(1): 9–14.

4 Stochetti, N., Maas, A.I.R. (2014) Traumatic intracranial hypertension. N Engl J Med; 370: 2121–30.

5 The Intensive Care Society. (2011) Guideline for the Transport of the Critically Ill Adult, 3rd edn. London: The Intensive Care Society.

6 Filonovsky, Y., Miller, P., Kao, J. (2010) Ketamine should not be used as an induction agent for intubation in patients with head injury. CJEM; 12(2): 154–7.

7 National Institute for Health and Care Excellence. (2014) Head Injury: Triage, Assessment, Investigation and Early Management of Head Injury in Infants, Children and Adults. Available at: http://www.nice.org.uk/guidance/CG176 (accessed November 2014).

8 Committee on Trauma of American College of Surgeons. (2012) *Advanced Trauma Life Support Provider Manual*, 9th edn. Chicago: Committee on Trauma of American College of Surgeons.

9 Dawes, R., Thomas, G.O.R. (2009) Battlefield resuscitation. Curr Opin Crit Care; 15(6): 527–35.

11.3 Cardiorespiratory failure

Gavin Perkins and Dermot McKeown

Objective

The objective of this section is to:

- Describe the indications, risks and technique for the intubation of patients with severe cardiorespiratory disease.

Introduction

Respiratory and cardiovascular emergencies are common indications for intubation in the emergency department. These patients generally require intubation because of failure to maintain adequate oxygenation and/or ventilation. Patients in extremis may need intubating for airway protection. The intubation process is identical to that described in Chapter 8.

Rapid sequence induction and intubation of patients with severe respiratory and/or cardiovascular disease is hazardous, with a greatly increased risk of complications during and after intubation. A reduced cardiac output and slower circulation time prolongs the onset and exaggerates the effects of drugs; i.e. there is increased sensitivity to the cardiorespiratory depressant effects of induction drugs. These patients have a low functional residual capacity (FRC) and therefore reduced oxygen reserve. Mechanical ventilation has a significant effect on the heart and lungs, including a reduction in venous return leading to a decreased cardiac output, and the risk of lung injury caused by high inspiratory volumes.

Rapidly obtain as much information as possible about the patient's past medical history and social circumstances before intubation; this may include information from hospital records, GP, relatives and carers. Many of these patients have acute exacerbations of a pre-existing illness, such as chronic obstructive pulmonary disease or chronic heart failure, or may be elderly with multiple comorbidities. Admission to an ICU may not be appropriate for some individuals and, whenever possible, early assessment by an intensivist is desirable.

Consider alternatives to intubation and ventilation, such as non-invasive ventilatory support. This is discussed further in Chapter 12. However, if intubation is indicated and significant collateral history is not available, the patient must be fully resuscitated immediately while awaiting further information.

Respiratory emergencies
Asthma

Indications for intubation: Consider intubation and invasive ventilation in any patient with asthma who is tiring, or where gas exchange continues to deteriorate (decreasing P_aO_2 or increasing P_aCO_2) despite optimal medical management. Follow the guidelines on the management of asthma published jointly by the British Thoracic Society (BTS) and Scottish Intercollegiate Guidelines Network (SIGN). All patients who have signs or symptoms of life-threatening asthma may potentially need intubation, especially those who have required ventilatory support before. Refer to the intensivist team if any of the following are present, even if intubation is not required immediately:

- deteriorating peak expiratory flow;
- persisting or worsening hypoxaemia;
- hypercapnoea;
- arterial blood gas analysis showing a worsening acidaemia;
- exhaustion, feeble respiration;
- drowsiness, confusion, altered conscious state;
- coma or respiratory arrest.

Standard therapy includes high-flow oxygen via a facemask with reservoir bag, continuous beta$_2$ agonist and an anticholinergic drug such as ipratropium by nebulizer, oral or intravenous steroids and intravenous magnesium.

Specific considerations during intubation: The patient will potentially be very difficult to pre-oxygenate because of hyperexpansion of the lungs and reduced ventilatory capacity. A reduced oxygen reserve makes the asthmatic patient prone to hypoxaemia during intubation. Give a rapid infusion of fluid before and during induction of anaesthesia: patients with acute severe asthma will be dehydrated. Stimulation of the larynx and trachea can provoke laryngospasm and bronchospasm. Once the tube has been placed in the trachea initiate ventilation carefully, with gentle inspiration and a long expiratory phase as the already hyperexpanded lung is vulnerable to further expansion causing volutrauma (with the risk of pneumothorax/tension pneumothorax) and potential cardiovascular collapse.

Ketamine: Ketamine is a potent bronchodilator and an excellent alternative to the standard induction drugs in patients with asthma. It has a relatively rapid onset intravenously: a dose of 1.5–2 mg kg^{-1} IV is used for induction. Peak concentrations are reached after one minute, and last for 10–15 minutes.

Use ketamine with caution in patients with ischaemic heart disease or hypertension, as it causes catecholamine release. It may also cause increased airway secretions, activation of pharyngeal reflexes and laryngospasm. Emergence phenomena are not usually a clinical problem in the emergency setting, but can be minimized with a small dose of benzodiazepine.

Post-intubation care: There are several specific considerations in the treatment of an asthmatic patient after intubation.

The expiratory airflow obstruction that occurs in patients with severe asthma may cause air trapping, evidenced by high airway pressures, and lung hyperinflation. This will generate significant intrinsic positive end expiratory pressure (PEEP$_i$ or auto-PEEP) and overdistension of alveoli, which increases intrathoracic pressure, reduces venous return and cardiac output, and causes hypotension. If this occurs, immediately disconnect the ventilator tubing from the tracheal tube and wait for complete exhalation: slow, steady chest compression may help to achieve adequate exhalation. The hypotension associated with auto-PEEP is exacerbated by hypovolaemia, which emphasizes the importance of fluid resuscitation before and immediately after RSI and intubation. Auto-PEEP is minimized by setting the ventilator to deliver the lowest minute volume that maintains oxygenation, and by providing a long expiratory time: providing the pH is above approximately 7.15 (H^+ 71 nmol L^{-1}), hypercarbia (permissive hypercapnia) is normally well tolerated. Asthmatic patients are at significant risk of developing tension pneumothoraces: these require immediate decompression. Any pneumothorax, whether under tension or not, will require insertion of a chest drain.

A bolus of a neuromuscular blocker such as rocuronium may be required to prevent the patient fighting the ventilator and further increasing airway pressure. Ensure that sedation is adequate. The addition of opioids will reduce respiratory drive, and are particularly useful when a strategy of permissive hypercapnia is used.

Mucous plugging occurs commonly in severe asthma: large plugs can occlude the tracheal tube, making it very difficult to ventilate the patient's lungs, and mucous plugging of the more distal airways can cause atelectasis, impairment of gas exchange and increased airway pressure. Therapeutic bronchoscopy may be necessary to remove large mucous plugs.

Chronic obstructive pulmonary disease (COPD)

The management principles for RSI and intubation of patients with COPD are similar to those with asthma.

Indications for intubation: Careful consideration as to whether invasive ventilation is appropriate should be made by a senior clinician, and ideally by the patient's respiratory specialist. Consider alternatives to IPPV, such as non-invasive ventilatory support, which reduces the need for intubation (see Chapter 12). Patients with COPD may require intubation if they are unable to clear secretions, protect their airway, continue to deteriorate despite non-invasive ventilatory support and medical therapy, or become apnoeic. NICE guidelines recommend that functional status, BMI, requirement for oxygen when stable, comorbidities and previous admissions to intensive care units should be considered, in addition to age and FEV_1, when assessing suitability for intubation and ventilation. Neither age nor FEV_1 should be used in isolation.

Considerations during intubation: By the time that patients with COPD require intubation they are often exhausted, have little oxygen reserve and are usually hypovolaemic. This makes them liable to arrhythmias and hypotension after intubation. A patient with COPD will require fluid loading and a reduced dose of induction drug for intubation. Normal doses of muscle relaxant are appropriate.

Post-intubation care: The potential complications and difficulties of positive pressure ventilation are the same for patients with COPD as they are for those with asthma.

Cardiovascular emergencies

Acute cardiogenic pulmonary oedema

Acute cardiogenic pulmonary oedema with respiratory failure is a relatively common medical emergency in the UK. The average UK emergency department will see between 50 and 100 of these patients per annum and, despite medical therapy and non-invasive ventilation, 5–7.5% will require intubation. Medical therapy includes high-flow oxygen via a mask with a reservoir bag, sublingual, buccal or intravenous nitrates, and consideration of intravenous loop diuretics. Continuous positive airway pressure (CPAP) is frequently effective; see Chapter 12.

Cardiogenic shock

These patients are critically ill and at significant risk of complications including cardiac arrest immediately after induction. Before intubation, it is often necessary to support the circulation with intravenous fluids and/or careful use of vasoactive drugs. If there is concomitant pulmonary oedema it may be difficult or impossible to pre-oxygenate adequately; furthermore, any induction drug may reduce cardiac output catastrophically. A carefully selected small dose of induction drug should be used, and may have to be omitted completely in patients in extremis; in these circumstances a small dose of midazolam (0.5–1 mg) will provide adequate sedation and amnesia for the intubation. In these patients, the circulation time for drugs is very prolonged. After intubation, avoid over ventilation because this will reduce venous return and cardiac output.

Dissection of the thoracic aorta or rupture of an abdominal aortic aneurysm

Unless absolutely necessary, avoid intubating in the emergency department patients with vascular emergencies such as dissection of the thoracic aorta or rupture of an abdominal aortic aneurysm. Intubation is best accomplished in the operating room with a scrubbed surgical team standing by. During intubation, the aim is to ablate the physiological response to laryngoscopy and intubation, and to prevent surges in blood pressure and heart rate. A pre-induction dose of an opioid such as fentanyl or alfentanil will reduce the sympathetic stimulation caused by laryngoscopy and intubation. Fentanyl is effective only if it is given at least three minutes before intubation, but be prepared to progress to intubation immediately if the patient becomes apnoeic.

Cardioversion

Patients who are physiologically compromised, or who have significant symptoms such as chest pain, with either a broad- or narrow-complex tachycardia may require electrical cardioversion. The initial management of these arrhythmias should follow European Resuscitation Council guidelines on peri-arrest arrhythmias. Electrical cardioversion is painful and therefore requires analgesia and sedation. There is no consensus on the best drugs to provide sedation or anaesthesia for cardioversion. Possibilities include carefully titrated doses of midazolam, propofol or etomidate; any of these can be combined with a short-acting opioid such as fentanyl or alfentanil.

These drugs provide a brief period of analgesia, sedation and subsequent amnesia during and after the procedure. In patients who have recently eaten, or who have significant gastro-oesophageal reflux, it may be preferable to undertake an RSI and intubation so that the airway is protected. If the patient has acute cardiogenic pulmonary oedema, or is shocked, follow the principles described in the preceding sections.

Sepsis

Patients who have severe sepsis or septic shock may exhibit respiratory distress because of their primary pathology and/or because of the compensatory increase in ventilation that accompanies a severe metabolic acidosis. After initial assessment using the ABCDE approach, ensure the sepsis six treatment bundle has been initiated (high-flow oxygen, blood cultures, broad-spectrum antibiotics, intravenous fluid challenges, serum lactate and haemoglobin, record accurate hourly urine output).

Indications for intubation remain as for all other conditions, but the patient will be in a precarious balance of high minute ventilation, marked reduction in vascular tone, and a variable cardiac output that is dependent on an adequate intravascular volume and heart rate.

Induction of anaesthesia, institution of positive pressure ventilation and attempts to deliver a minute ventilation sufficient to compensate for severe metabolic acidosis are likely to precipitate cardiovascular collapse.

Early involvement of the intensive care team is essential: invasive arterial and central venous pressure monitoring, vasopressors and inotropes may all be required before RSI. Consider using ketamine as the induction drug to minimize the risk of worsening hypotension. Etomidate causes adrenocortical suppression; it should be avoided in sepsis.

Anaphylaxis and angio-oedema

Anaphylaxis to any allergen may lead to upper airway obstruction caused by severe oedema. Generally, this initially affects the eyelids, face and lips and makes intubation very difficult.

Early use of adrenaline frequently prevents progression of this condition, but if the patient continues to deteriorate a judgement may have to be made by a senior practitioner to proceed with intubation.

Laryngeal and pharyngeal oedema develop more slowly, but may make it difficult to see the larynx and necessitate intubation with a smaller tracheal tube. Tissues are swollen and friable, so that minor trauma may increase the swelling: gentle use of instruments is essential. These patients have many characteristics that lead to the 'can't intubate, can't oxygenate' situation and a clear plan for failed intubation with all appropriate backup devices and personnel must be immediately available. Even if the airway is controlled, there may be marked bronchospasm and treatment will be similar to that for severe asthma.

Even though facial swelling may quickly resolve, do not remove the tracheal tube until an audible inspiratory leak at low pressure is evident when the cuff is deflated: by this stage the patient will be in an intensive care unit. As with the management of patients with facial burns, the tracheal tube should not be cut and attention should be paid to tube ties, which may become tighter if swelling continues.

Although the aetoiology of angio-oedema is entirely different to anaphylaxis, it shares a necessity to assess, and where appropriate, manage the airway as an early priority.

Summary

- There are many cardiorespiratory emergencies requiring urgent induction of anaesthesia and intubation.
- A reduced reservoir of oxygen and impaired cardiovascular reserve amplify the side effects of anaesthetic and sedative drugs.
- Intensive care specialists must be involved at an early stage and, whenever possible, before intubation.
- The dose of induction drugs must be modified carefully to reflect the patient's physiological state: vasoactive drugs will probably be required.
- Conversion from spontaneous to positive pressure ventilation may cause cardiovascular decompensation.

Acknowledgement

This chapter has been updated from the first edition chapter, which was written by Alasdair Gray and Dermot McKeown.

Further reading

1   British Thoracic Society and Scottish Intercollegiate Guidelines Network. (2008) *British Guideline on the Management of Asthma. A National Clinical Guideline.* London: British Thoracic Society and Scottish Intercollegiate Guidelines Network. Available at: www.sign.ac.uk (accessed November 2014).

2   National Institute for Health and Clinical Excellence. (2010) *Clinical Guideline 101. Chronic Obstructive Pulmonary Disease. Management of Chronic Obstructive Pulmonary Disease in Adults in Primary and Secondary Care (partial update 2010).* London: National Institute for Health and Clinical Excellence. Available at: http://guidance.nice.org.uk/CG101/NICEGuidance/pdf/English (accessed November 2014).

3   Dellinger, R.P., Levy, M.M., Rhodes, A. *et al.*; Surviving Sepsis Campaign Guidelines Committee including the Pediatric Subgroup. (2013) Surviving Sepsis Campaign: international guidelines for management of severe sepsis and septic shock: 2012. Crit Care Med; 41: 580–637.

4   McLean-Tooke, A.P.C., Bethune, C.A., Fay, A.C., Spickett, G.P. (2003) Adrenaline in the treatment of anaphylaxis: what is the evidence? BMJ; 327: 1332–5.

5   Resuscitation Council (UK). (2008) *Emergency Treatment of Anaphylactic Reactions.* London: Resuscitation Council (UK). Available at: www.resus.org.uk/pages/reaction.pdf (accessed November 2014).

11.4 Non-traumatic coma and seizures

Carl Gwinnutt

Objectives

The objectives of this section are to:

- Understand the immediate risks to the comatose or convulsing patient.
- Understand the principles of immediate airway management in these patients.
- Be familiar with the modifications to advanced airway techniques needed in the special circumstances of non-traumatic coma and seizures.
- Understand what these modifications mean, in practical terms, for the emergency airway practitioner.
- Be aware of the pitfalls frequently encountered in these patients.

Introduction

Coma is the result of either (a) diffuse, generalized inhibition of brain function (e.g. drugs, hypoglycaemia) or (b) disturbance of the brainstem, which can be direct (e.g. tumour) or indirect (e.g. haematoma, hydrocephalus), causing inhibition of the reticular activating system. As a result, there is a state of unconsciousness with no reaction to external or internal stimuli, but there is preservation of some reflex activity. The Glasgow Coma Scale (GCS) score, although originally devised for use in head-injured patients, is frequently used to define coma (as a score of 8 or less). The emergency airway management of patients with traumatic coma is described earlier in this chapter, in the trauma and raised intracranial pressure section. This section focuses on the emergency airway management of patients with non-traumatic coma and seizures. As an aide-memoire some of the common causes of non-traumatic coma are listed in Box 11.2, using the mnemonic COMA. However, there is often a combination of causes: a patient with alcohol intoxication who has fallen may also have an extradural haematoma.

Risks to the comatose or convulsing patient

Because comatose patients have altered brainstem neuronal activity, there is attenuation of respiratory function, vasomotor tone and protective laryngeal reflexes. Therefore, the most significant risks faced by these patients are hypoxaemia, hypercarbia, cardiac arrhythmias, hypotension and aspiration of gastric contents. Some patients, particularly those with generalized brain dysfunction, may also have grand mal seizures because of loss of normal inhibitory influences. If prolonged, these may result in rhabdomyolysis,

---

Box 11.2 Causes of non-traumatic coma (mnemonic: COMA)

Cerebral:
- Tumour
- Infection: meningitis, encephalitis, cerebral abscess
- Cerebral haemorrhage: extra/subdural, intracerebral, subarachnoid
- Cerebral/cerebellar ischaemia, infarction
- Post-ictal
- Hydrocephalus

Overdose:
- Alcohol, and alcohol withdrawal
- Drugs: opioids, sedatives, hypnotics, salicylates

Metabolic/endocrine:
- Diabetic emergencies: hypoglycaemia or hyperglycaemia
- Electrolyte disturbances: sodium, calcium and magnesium
- Organ failure: renal, hepatic, pulmonary, cardiac
- Thyroid, adrenal, pituitary dysfunction
- Hypothermia, hyperthermia

Airway/asphyxia:
- Hypoxaemia
- Hypercapnoea

hyperthermia and further brain injury, secondary to severe hypoxaemia and metabolic acidosis.

Immediate treatment principles

Establish and maintain a patent airway and give high-concentration oxygen. For some comatose patients, simple airway manoeuvres (chin lift or jaw thrust), basic adjuncts (oropharyngeal and/or nasopharyngeal airways), high-flow oxygen via a facemask with reservoir bag, and close observation may be all that is necessary. Examples of such patients include those with hypoglycaemia or an opioid overdose before specific treatment is given. In an epileptic patient with a self-limiting grand mal seizure, airway protection from aspiration is rarely required because the uncoordinated motor activity precludes coordinated expulsion of gastric contents, and protective laryngeal reflexes return early during the recovery phase. Positioning the patient on their side on a tipping trolley, suctioning secretions and blood, the application of a jaw thrust or insertion of a nasopharyngeal airway to relieve obstruction by the tongue are usually all that is necessary.

Where hypoventilation occurs in a patient with non-traumatic coma, ventilation using a bag-mask device may be necessary to maintain oxygenation and prevent hypercarbia, before securing a definitive airway. Whether the person performing this task possesses the skills necessary to secure a definitive airway or not, it will also effectively begin the process of pre-oxygenation before RSI and intubation, maximizing the patient's chances of a good outcome.

While managing the airway, consider the possible causes of the underlying coma. At best it may be reversible, or it may be possible to improve the level of consciousness, thereby avoiding the need to intubate. The underlying cause may influence the technique used for securing the airway.

Obtain as much history about the patient as is feasible given the clinical circumstances. For example:

- Sudden collapse with coma implies a neurovascular cause (ischaemic or haemorrhagic stroke, subarachnoid haemorrhage) or cardiac arrhythmia;
- Gradual deterioration (minutes to a few hours) into coma is associated more frequently with metabolic causes and drug intoxication;
- Deterioration into coma over a longer period is more usually associated with infection and organ failure (hepatic, respiratory, renal or endocrine);
- Evidence of drug overdose is often found at the scene. Seek information from pre-hospital personnel wherever possible;
- Consider raised ICP in any patient who has a non-traumatic cause of reduced consciousness;
- Remain vigilant to the possibilty of intracranial infection since this is an easily missed and time-critical diagnosis.

> **Box 11.3 Signs of raised intracranial pressure**
>
> - Reduced consciousness
> - Irregular or slow respiratory pattern
> - Hypertension and bradycardia
> - Extensor posturing
> - Papilloedema
> - Pupillary signs

Further confirmatory signs of an increased ICP may also be apparent in the rapid initial assessment of the comatose or seizing patient (Box 11.3). In these circumstances techniques to reduce the pressor response to laryngoscopy and intubation will form part of the RSI.

The urgency of the situation may preclude a full physical examination and a rapid initial assessment may be all that can be achieved before securing a definitive airway. In these circumstances the full general examination is deferred until the airway is secured.

All comatose patients must have their capillary or venous glucose and temperature measured; take an arterial blood sample if time permits. This frequently provides information that will inform the immediate management plan and act as a baseline against which further results can be compared.

Indications for intubation in the non-traumatic coma or convulsing patient

Determining when to proceed from supportive airway measures to intubation is one of the key challenges clinicians face when managing patients in coma of non-traumatic origin, or those who are seizing. As a general rule the decision to intubate is made when the risks of not intervening outweigh the risks of doing so. Clinical experience aids the decision-making process. Box 11.4 lists the absolute and relative indications for securing a definitive airway in these patients.

There is no clear guideline that defines specifically the duration of generalized seizure activity before there is a need to intubate the patient. In UK practice, most experienced clinicians would consider tracheal intubation in those patients with seizures lasting more than 15 minutes following hospital arrival, and refractory to first-line anticonvulsant therapy (benzodiazepines). In patients with an established diagnosis of epilepsy, second-line anticonvulsant therapy is usually commenced (e.g. phenytoin) before intubation. When there is no previous history of seizures the need for CT scanning of the head usually brings forward the decision to intubate.

Box 11.4 Indications for tracheal intubation in non-traumatic coma and seizures

Failure to maintain a patent airway:
- Obstruction despite the use of basic manoeuvres and adjuncts
- Lack of protective laryngeal reflexes
- Seizures refractory to treatment, compromising the airway

Failure of ventilation:
- Apnoea
- Hypoxaemia ($S_pO_2 < 92\%$, $P_aO_2 < 8$ kPa) on supplemental oxygen (60%)
- Hypercapnoea ($P_aCO_2 > 6.5$ kPa)

Prolonged seizure activity:
- Includes generalized status epilepticus, refractory to anticonvulsant treatment

To facilitate treatment of the underlying condition:
- Intracranial haemorrhage with raised ICP
- Tricyclic antidepressant overdose with a metabolic acidosis and/or GCS <9
- High-risk patients who require CT scanning
- Patients who require transportation

The technique of tracheal intubation

The comatose patient

Although it may be physically possible to intubate the comatose patient without using drugs, this is seldom advisable. Intubating conditions will be far from ideal, and apart from the risk of trauma and laryngospasm, autonomic reflex activity will cause an increase in blood pressure and ICP. Either or both of these may worsen the underlying cause of coma or precipitate further complications, for example:

- Hypertension may cause further bleeding after an intracranial haemorrhage.
- A rise in ICP may cause coning.

Rapid sequence induction is, therefore, the technique of choice for securing the airway in this group of patients with the following considerations.

Pre-oxygenation

Pre-existing hypoxaemia ($P_aO_2 < 8$ kPa, 60 mmHg) will cause an increase in cerebral blood flow and ICP, and may also be contributing to the decreased level of consciousness. If the patient's spontaneous ventilatory efforts are severely impaired, pre-oxygenation will require assisted ventilation. Use small tidal volumes and low inflation pressures to avoid gastric distension and an increased risk of regurgitation.

Cricoid pressure

Application of cricoid pressure is indicated because there may not have been time for the stomach to empty before the onset of coma, and many causes of coma delay gastric emptying, e.g. opioids, salicylate poisoning, hypoxaemia, hyperglycaemia, hypothermia, increased ICP.

Drugs for induction of anaesthesia

Propofol (used most commonly) and thiopental sodium are suitable for use in comatose patients. Ketamine may also be considered. A reduced dose will be required, when coma is drug induced or in the presence of hypovolaemia.

Neuromuscular blocking drugs

Suxamethonium remains the drug of choice in most cases, but high-dose rocuronium may be considered by an experienced practitioner familiar with its use. The use of suxamethonium has been questioned when the ICP is known to be high, but when given with an anaesthetic induction drug, suxamethonium causes a negligible increase in ICP.

Adjuvant treatment

Intravenous opioids given before the induction of anaesthesia will attenuate the autonomic reflexes that cause an increase in blood pressure and ICP. The opioids most commonly used are fentanyl and alfentanil, given one to three minutes before laryngoscopy (see Chapter 8).

The convulsing patient

The motor manifestations of seizures can be stopped and muscle relaxation achieved to facilitate tracheal intubation by giving neuromuscular blocking drugs alone. This is totally inappropriate as neuronal seizure activity will continue and the patient could be harmed by the cardiovascular response to intubation. Furthermore, once the seizures stop, there is a risk of the patient becoming aware while still paralyzed. Consequently, general anaesthesia is required and both an intravenous induction drug and a neuromuscular blocking drug must be given. Patients who are fitting may have vomited or bitten their lips or tongue: there may be vomit or blood in the airway that will make intubation more difficult. Ensure that a wide-bore rigid sucker (e.g. Yankauer) is always immediately available. The technique of tracheal intubation follows that described in Chapter 8, with the following additional considerations.

Pre-oxygenation

This may be difficult to achieve because of uncoordinated respiratory effort and myoclonus of the upper airway, oropharynx and muscles of mastication. An attempt should be made, even if it is only possible to apply high-flow oxygen to the patient's mouth and nose. Because of this potential difficulty, time to desaturation during the initial intubation attempt may be short. Apnoeic oxygenation may be particularly useful in this situation.

Drugs for the induction of anaesthesia

Thiopental sodium has profound anticonvulsant activity and will terminate most seizures at the dose used to induce unconsciousness. It also causes marked myocardial depression, and therefore a reduced dose may be required in some circumstances. Although propofol may cause myoclonic activity, it has anticonvulsant properties and is an acceptable alternative. Patients with focal seizures rarely require emergency airway management.

Adjuvant treatment

The same considerations apply as for the comatose patient. Once ventilation is established, aim for P_aO_2 12–15 kPa and a P_aCO_2 4.6–5.3 kPa.

Pitfalls

1. Failure to recognize and treat hypoglycaemia, opioid overdose or intracranial infection.
2. Failure to recognize the importance of the anticipated clinical course. This is particularly true in cases of deliberate poisoning with tricyclic antidepressants, anticonvulsants and antiarrhythmics. By considering the pharmacodynamic and pharmacokinetic profiles of the ingested substance, and an approximate time of ingestion, it is possible to predict with reasonable certainty when the clinical state of the patient is likely to worsen. Early intervention, including intubation and ventilation with intensive care support, when the patient is more tolerant of the cardiovascular side effects of the drugs used, is preferable to acting later in an increasingly unstable patient.
3. A sedated patient may have subclinical seizure activity (e.g. non-convulsive status epilepticus), the clinical maifestations of which are suppressed either by sedation or paralysis. Neurophysiological assessment is important in identifying these patients and preventing avoidable brain injury.
4. The intubated, paralyzed patient can still be fitting, and will therefore require effective sedation; an infusion of propofol (2–12 mg kg^{-1} h^{-1}), thiopental (2–5 mg kg^{-1} h^{-1}) or midazolam (0.05–0.5 mg kg^{-1} h^{-1}) can be used along with anticonvulsants. Whilst high infusion rates of these drugs may be required to stop seizure activity, this can result in significant accumulation and toxicity and should therefore be used for short periods

of time (1–2 hours) wherever possible, by which time other anti-epileptic medication may have become effective. Continuous bedside EEG may facilitate accurate management of seizures by enabling monitoring of seizure activity and response to treatment. In most cases it will be necessary to allow motor recovery to occur to assess the response to anticonvulsant treatment. In the sedated, paralyzed patient, bursts of hypertension, tachycardia and pupillary dilatation are suggestive of seizure activity.

5. New prolonged seizure activity usually represents a significant change in seizure behaviour for the patient. Look for an underlying cause (e.g. metabolic, infective, cerebrovascular event).

Summary

- Patients who are in coma of a non-traumatic origin, or fitting, often present specific problems to the airway practitioner.
- The method for securing a definitive airway in these patients is modified according to the particular circumstances of each case.
- Early recognition of the high risk of these patients, awareness of the potential pitfalls and a team-based approach will maximize the chances of obtaining a good patient outcome.

Acknowledgement

This chapter has been updated from the first edition chapter, which was written by Neil Robinson and Carl Gwinnutt.

Further reading

1 Huff, J.S., Morris, D.L., Kothari, R.U., Gibbs, M. A.; Emergency Medicine Seizure Study Group. (2001) Emergency department management of patients with seizures: a multicenter study. Acad Emerg Med; 8: 622–8.

2 Gwinnutt,C., Carroll, C., Sebastian, J. (2012) Neurological emergencies. In Nolan J. Soar J. (eds.), *Anaesthesia for Emergency Care*. Oxford: Oxford University Press.

11.5 Pre-hospital care

Jonathan Benger

Objectives

The objectives of this section are to understand:

- The background and principles of pre-hospital RSI and tracheal intubation.
- The differences between in-hospital and pre-hospital RSI, and the potential problems that are unique to this environment.

Background

The procedure of pre-hospital RSI is carried out throughout most of Europe. In the UK, it is carried out only by doctors working in pre-hospital care, and relatively infrequently. Worldwide, pre-hospital intubation is carried out in several ways by a variety of practitioners. The procedure is performed with and without drugs. When drugs are used they may consist of a benzodiazepine only or an induction drug with a neuromuscular blocking drug. Practitioners include paramedics, nurses and doctors. Paramedics have markedly different experience and training in different systems. Doctors need to be aware of the possible indications for pre-hospital RSI and the potential hazards of the procedure outside the usual hospital environment.

Pre-hospital rapid sequence induction in an emergency medical service

Pre-hospital RSI should not be undertaken by individuals working in isolation; it should be part of a well-organized system, with integral clinical governance. A system supporting the procedure needs to provide the following elements:

- A structure to ensure that practitioners are competent to perform the procedure.
- Control, support and supervision of practitioners.
- Training and continuing education.
- Standard guidelines or protocols.
- Techniques and equipment that bring the procedure as close as possible to standards achieved in hospital (e.g. national standards of anaesthetic monitoring).
- Audit and quality assurance programmes.

Indications

The *possible* indications for pre-hospital RSI are essentially the same as for RSI in the emergency department. These are discussed comprehensively in Chapter 4. In every case a rapid but thorough on-scene risk/benefit assessment is made, and the potential benefits of pre-hospital RSI are balanced against the risks of the procedure in a given scenario. Examples of factors influencing the decision might include the experience of the practitioner, assistance available, the time to hospital, the effect of basic airway manoeuvres, expected clinical course or anticipated difficulties with the procedure (e.g. an anticipated difficult intubation).

While some situations will require little consideration (e.g. where gross hypoxaemia exists despite basic airway manoeuvres, and airway reflexes prevent non-drug assisted intubation), in others the potential benefit may be less clear.

Principles

1. Patients in near or actual cardiorespiratory arrest, where airway reflexes are lost, may be intubated without drugs, following simple airway manoeuvres and bag-mask ventilation.
2. The only absolute indication for pre-hospital RSI is total failure to establish a patent airway by any other means, in a patient who requires drug administration to counter airway reflexes. This is an extremely rare event.
3. In all other cases, the potential benefits of RSI must be weighed against the potential risks. Pre-hospital practitioners work in a highly exposed situation, and RSI requires significant time, which may exceed the journey time to the nearest hospital.
4. In general, if the airway is adequate, pre-hospital RSI is not required. Exceptions might be a prolonged transport time, or where the anticipated clinical course is one of rapid deterioration (e.g. airway burns).

Technique

Key considerations in the technique of pre-hospital RSI:
- Safety
- Patient access
- Patient positioning
- Environment
- Equipment
- Assistance

Safety

As in all pre-hospital care, safety is of paramount importance. Safety considerations extend to the practitioner, colleagues on scene and the patient(s). RSI should not be undertaken in an area that is, or may become, unsafe. This may require the patient to be moved before RSI.

Patient access

Good patient access is essential, particularly if difficulties are encountered. It is helpful to consider what will happen if a surgical airway is required. In general, it is not appropriate to attempt intubation before extrication (e.g. from a crashed vehicle) unless all other attempts to maintain the airway have failed: in the vast majority of cases airway intervention should be restricted to simple manoeuvres and provision of oxygen until extrication and full patient access can be achieved. Give drugs to trapped or inaccessible persons only with extreme caution since these may precipitate deterioration in a previously adequate airway, which cannot then be restored. While RSI may be undertaken in an ambulance, there is a risk of compromising both access and positioning because of the relatively cramped conditions. This must be balanced against the weather protection and light that are provided within a vehicle.

Patient positioning

It is difficult to intubate a patient lying on the floor or on their side: in general, the practitioner will have to lie prone. In some circumstances, such as where gross hypoxaemia exists despite basic airway manoeuvres, there may be little alternative. Where possible, move the patient to a more convenient height, usually onto an ambulance trolley. Ensure that all equipment remains readily to hand; if this is laid out on the floor then the patient should be at a height where a kneeling practitioner can comfortably intubate.

Environment

Sunlight will cause the practitioner's pupils to constrict, making subsequent laryngoscopy very difficult: the patient and practitioner should therefore be shaded for the procedure. Conversely, the patient will become very cold in a wet or wintry environment, particularly following intubation and paralysis. Beware of groups of curious bystanders, friends or relations: they can become interfering or hostile, particularly if things do not seem to be going well.

Equipment

Much of the equipment taken for granted in hospitals is either not available or less reliable in the pre-hospital environment. Ensure that adequate oxygen, suction and monitoring (including waveform capnography) are available, and that everything that might be required (including surgical airway equipment) is available and fully functional. Colourimetric carbon dioxide detectors, which provide visual confirmation of carbon dioxide with the first breath following intubation, are valuable, but do not replace the need for waveform capnography. Videolaryngoscopes are beginning to be used in pre-hospital intubation, but their utility has yet to be established. Such devices need to be robust, reliable and weather-proof, and indirect visualization may be hampered by blood and secretions in the airway, as well as the climatic conditions. For this reason direct laryngoscopy remains an essential skill for pre-hospital practitioners.

Assistance

Skilled assistance is often less readily available, particularly in pre-hospital systems where RSI and tracheal intubation is not commonplace. Rapid sequence induction should be undertaken only with trained assistance. Additional people may also be required to provide skills such as manual stabilization of the cervical spine.

Summary

- Pre-hospital RSI and tracheal intubation should be carried out only in an organized and governed system.
- Each pre-hospital RSI and intubation should be performed only after a risk/benefit assessment.
- The indications for pre-hospital RSI and tracheal intubation are similar to those in hospital, but their application will depend upon several factors that are specific to each situation. These include the experience of the practitioner, assistance available, the transport time to hospital, the patient's condition and anticipated clinical course.
- The practitioner must be familiar with the unique aspects of pre-hospital care and experienced in RSI and tracheal intubation before undertaking this procedure.

Acknowledgement

This chapter has been updated from the first edition chapter, which was written by David Lockey and Jonathan Benger.

Further reading

1   Association of Anaesthetists of Great Britain and Ireland. (2009) *AAGBI Safety Guideline: Pre-Hospital Anaesthesia.* London: AAGBI. Available at: http://www.aagbi.org/sites/default/files/prehospital_glossy09.pdf (accessed January 2015).

2. Lossius, H.M., Røislien, J., Lockey, D.J. (2012) Patient safety in pre-hospital emergency tracheal intubation: a comprehensive meta-analysis of the intubation success rates of EMS providers. Crit Care; 16: R24. Available at: http://ccforum.com/content/pdf/cc11189.pdf (accessed January 2015).

11.6 The pregnant patient

John Clift

Objectives

The objectives of this section are to:

- Understand the important considerations when managing an obstetric airway.
- Be able to describe the management options specific to obstetrics.
- Consider the approach to failed intubation in the obstetric patient.

Introduction

The airway of the obstetric patient is particularly challenging, as evidenced by the increased rate of failed intubation compared with the non-obstetric patient. In this unique situation there are two patients to consider, and optimizing the condition of the mother usually results in the best conditions for the fetus.

Special considerations in the obstetric patient

Physiological

Supine hypotensive syndrome occurs from mid-pregnancy and is caused by the gravid uterus compressing the inferior vena cava. This reduces venous return and cardiac output, which can cause maternal hypotension and placental hypoperfusion. It is best avoided by using a left lateral tilt of 30° if on a table that can tilt, or using a wedge placed under the right hip.

At term there is a 20% reduction in functional residual capacity (FRC) of the lungs and a 20% increase in oxygen consumption. The clinical implication of this is that after the onset of apnoea the patient's arterial blood desaturates much quicker than in the non-gravid state. A full 3 minutes pre-oxygenation with high-flow oxygen is essential before inducing anaesthesia.

The reduction in lower oesophageal sphincter pressure (due to progesterone) and elevated intra-abdominal pressure (due to the gravid uterus) increase the risk of reflux and aspiration of gastric contents. Gastric emptying is normal in pregnancy but is prolonged with opiates and with labour. The patient is at increased risk of aspiration from 16 weeks gestation or earlier if she has symptoms of reflux. From this stage, the need for anaesthesia will necessitate a rapid sequence induction (RSI) and consideration of antacid prophylaxis. Once the baby is delivered the risk returns to non-pregnant levels within 24–48 hours after delivery, except where symptoms of reflux persist.

Anatomical

There are many anatomical factors that contribute to an increased risk of failed intubation in an obstetric patient. These include:

- full dentition;
- increase in oedema of larynx and pharynx, which may be more pronounced in pre-eclampsia/eclampsia;
- large breasts;
- increase in chest wall diameter;
- increase in fatty tissue.

All of these make it more difficult to insert the laryngoscope and see the vocal cords.

Pharmacology specific to the obstetric patient

The pharmacology for RSI is discussed in Chapter 7; however, there are considerations that are specific to the obstetric patient.

To reduce gastric content acidity and its effects on the lungs if aspirated, antacid prophylaxis is usually given. Most commonly an H_2 receptor blocker such as ranitidine (two oral doses of 150 mg 12 hours apart) is given. In an emergency this is given intravenously in a dose of 50 mg. Oral sodium citrate 30 mL 0.3 M is given immediately before induction and will provide immediate protection, but its effects are short-lived.

RSI is performed because of the risk of aspiration of gastric contents. The most common induction drug is thiopental sodium 5 mg kg^{-1} although etomidate or ketamine may be used in the shocked patient. Suxamethonium 1.5 mg kg^{-1} is the muscle relaxant of choice for intubation, although rocuronium may also be considered.

Rapid sequence induction and tracheal intubation

This is performed as previously described in Chapter 8, with the following modifications.

The head elevated or 'ramp' position may make intubation easier, particularly in an obese individual. Large breasts and use of cricoid pressure may make it difficult to insert the laryngoscope blade – use of a polio blade or short handled Macintosh laryngoscope may make this easier. A McCoy laryngoscope may improve the view of the glottis.

Failed intubation and failed ventilation

The risk of failed intubation in the obstetric population may be as frequent as 1 in 300, compared to a background rate of 1 in 2000 in the non-obstetric population. This is for the anatomical and physiological reasons described previously and other factors such as:

- stress caused by the perceived urgency to induce anaesthesia;
- incorrect application of cricoid pressure;
- operator lack of experience because fewer caesarean sections are performed under general anaesthesia;
- left lateral tilt;
- the increase in the number of obese pregnant patients.

Failure to intubate, and in particular oxygenate, is potentially life-threatening to mother and baby. It requires early recognition and management by expedient progression through a well-rehearsed drill.

Careful assessment of the airway before attempting RSI and tracheal intubation may enable identification of a difficult airway and appropriate preparation before induction. The management of the difficult or failed airway is discussed in Chapter 9.

Particular points relevant to the obstetric patient are:

- CALL FOR HELP early.
- Do not give a second dose of suxamethonium.
- Maintain cricoid pressure and keep mother supine with left lateral uterine displacement.
- Maternal oxygenation is the first priority and takes preference over concerns about the fetus or the risk of regurgitation.
- If the patient begins to breathe at any point, turn her to the left lateral position.

Once the patient is oxygenated, the urgency of the procedure is then considered.

Whether to wake or continue?

The decision whether to wake the patient once oxygenation has been achieved will depend on the clinical circumstances and the means by which oxygenation has been achieved.

The situation can be considered in the context of:

1. Failed intubation following RSI for non-obstetric reasons in the pregnant patient.
2. Failed intubation following induction of anaesthesia for obstetric surgery (usually operative delivery).

In non-obstetric emergencies involving the pregnant patient, the option to wake the patient will often not apply because the decision to intubate will not have been taken lightly and allowing the patient to wake may not prove practical or possible. This may not be the case for obstetric surgery, even obstetric emergencies, depending on whether the nature of the emergency poses a risk to the mother or to the baby.

In the context of surgery, if, despite being difficult, the airway has been secured by means of an orotracheal tube and there are no ongoing concerns about the patency or security of the airway, surgery can continue. However, where the airway is less well protected or the security of the airway is suboptimal (e.g. mask ventilation, supraglottic airway device or surgical airway), the situation will need to be carefully assessed.

A patient being anaesthetized for an elective caesarean section should be awoken and either a different anaesthetic technique or different method of securing the airway used. The patient undergoing general anaesthesia for operative control of life-threatening bleeding should remain anaesthetized to enable the surgery to continue without delay. Occasionally, the decision to continue may be unclear, such as in the case of a compromised fetus. Senior decision-making is required for these situations.

Pre-eclampsia

Pre-eclampsia merits special mention because of the problems associated with airway management. If possible, avoid general anaesthesia in these patients. If general anaesthesia must proceed, consider the following:

1. The increased incidence of difficult intubation because of oedema of the upper airway.

2. The increased risk of intracranial haemorrhage, associated with surges in blood pressure, in the pre-eclamptic or hypertensive obstetric patient. Intracranial haemorrhage is the most frequent cause of serious morbidity and mortality in the pre-eclamptic patient. Before induction reduce the blood pressure to less than 160/100 mmHg and ideally less than 150/90 mmHg. Obtund the pressor response to intubation by injecting alfentanil (10 mcg kg^{-1}) before giving the induction drug. For caesarean section, inform the paediatrician that opiates have been given because they may cause neonatal sedation and respiratory depression. Alternative drugs that can be given as a slow bolus to obtund the hypertensive response to laryngoscopy include labetalol (10–20 mg) and magnesium (40 mg kg^{-1}).

Training

Practitioners should take up opportunities to participate in providing elective general anaesthesia for the obstetric patient where this is indicated, because the preference for regional anaesthesia for operative delivery means that these learning opportunities are much less common.

An alternative training option, available to all specialties, is the use of simulation training. High-fidelity simulation sessions provide an excellent forum for learning and reinforcing the management of specific scenarios, including the management of the difficult or failed obstetric airway.

Summary

- There are several physiological and anatomical factors which make the obstetric airway more difficult to manage than that of the non-obstetric population.
- Training opportunities are becoming rarer and there is an increased reliance on simulation.
- The operator must know a simple, well-rehearsed failed intubation drill.
- The primary goal is to maintain oxygenation of the mother.

Further reading

1 Clift, J. (2008) Maternal physiology and obstetrics. In Heazell, A., Clift, J. (eds.), *Obstetrics for Anaesthetists*. Cambridge: Cambridge University Press.

2 Rucklidge, M., Hinton, C. (2012) Difficult and failed intubation in obstetrics. Cont Educ Anaesthesia Crit Care Pain; 12(2): 86–91.

Chapter 12	Non-invasive ventilatory support
	Dinendra S. Gill and Gavin Perkins

Objectives

The objectives of this chapter are to understand:

- The mechanisms of action of non-invasive ventilation.
- The clinical applications for non-invasive ventilation in the acute setting.
- The role of continuous positive airway pressure (CPAP) versus non-invasive positive pressure ventilation (NIPPV).
- The limitations and complications of non-invasive ventilation.
- The practical application of non-invasive ventilation.

Introduction

Non-invasive ventilation (NIV) is the umbrella term used to describe the provision of ventilatory support through the patient's upper airway using a mask or similar device. NIV is principally indicated in patients with chronic obstructive pulmonary disease (COPD) with respiratory distress and hypercapnia, and in acute cardiogenic pulmonary oedema. Evidence indicates a reduction in intubation rates and mortality, particularly in patients with COPD. NIV may also be used in patients who are not considered suitable for intubation. A ceiling of treatment, and whether escalation to intubation is indicated, must be defined at the outset. Do not use NIV as a substitute for intubation and invasive ventilation if the latter is more appropriate. Early consultation with the intensive care team is imperative in both cases.

Modes of non-invasive ventilation

The terminology used to describe different types of NIV is complex. Outside the intensive care unit the two main types of NIV used in the UK are:

Emergency Airway Management, Second Edition, ed. Andrew Burtenshaw, Jonathan Benger and Jerry Nolan. Published by Cambridge University Press. © College of Emergency Medicine, London, 2015.

- Continuous positive airway pressure (CPAP). During CPAP a constant positive pressure is applied throughout the respiratory cycle.
- Non-invasive positive pressure ventilation (NIPPV). NIPPV provides wo levels of pressure support during the ventilator cycle – one during expiration and a higher one during inspiration.

Mechanisms of action

Continuous positive airway pressure

CPAP is typically used to correct hypoxaemia in type 1 respiratory failure (P_aO_2 < 8 kPa with a normal or low P_aCO_2). It has several mechanisms of action:

- Increase in functional residual capacity (FRC) – the volume of gas remaining in the lungs at the end of a normal expiration. A low FRC causes atelectasis and lung collapse, leading to ventilation/perfusion ($\dot{V}/\dot{Q}$) mismatch, reduced pulmonary compliance and increased airway resistance. This increases the work of breathing. Restoration of the FRC towards normal improves oxygenation and reduces work of breathing.
- Reopening closed or under-ventilated alveoli (recruitment). This occurs as part of the general improvement in FRC and reduces intrapulmonary shunting (perfusion of unventilated alveoli), thereby improving oxygenation.
- Reduction in left ventricular transmural pressure. This is of value in left ventricular failure, and may be the main mechanism by which CPAP improves oxygenation in acute cardiogenic pulmonary oedema. It also reduces afterload and preload, to which the failing heart is sensitive. CPAP does not drive pulmonary oedema fluid back into the circulation, and total lung water may not change despite clinical improvement.
- Reducing threshold work. In patients with auto-PEEP (intrinsic positive end expiratory pressure) or dynamic hyperinflation, the inspiratory muscles have to work to drop the alveolar pressure from its positive, end expiratory value to less than the upper airway pressure (normally zero) before inspiratory gas flow occurs. This is termed threshold work, and may be significant. By increasing the airway pressure, CPAP reduces the work required to initiate inspiratory flow. This may reduce respiratory rate and P_aCO_2, and is the reason that CPAP is sometimes considered to provide ventilatory support as well as correction of hypoxaemia.
- Airway splinting. CPAP is a specific treatment for obstructive sleep apnoea, and is often of value in patients with temporary airway problems.

- Delivery of high F_iO_2. Efficient CPAP systems deliver oxygen at flows that exceed the patient's peak inspiratory flow, without rebreathing; thus the selected inspired oxygen concentration (up to 100%) is delivered reliably.

Non-invasive positive pressure ventilation

NIPPV is a combination of CPAP with pressure support. Two pressure settings are selected: a higher, inspiratory positive airway pressure (IPAP), and a lower, expiratory positive airway pressure (EPAP). The difference between them generates a tidal volume (ventilation). EPAP is effectively CPAP – it recruits under-ventilated alveoli and increases FRC (improving oxygenation), and reduces threshold work in the presence of auto-PEEP (see above). When the patient is breathing spontaneously, the patient's respiratory effort triggers both the inspiratory and expiratory phase of the respiratory cycle. In the basic form of this mode, if the patient develops apnoea, no respiratory assistance will occur; however, many NIPPV machines incorporate a backup rate of 6–8 breaths per minute. In timed mode, mandatory breaths are delivered, although patient triggering is also possible. Use of NIPPV decreases respiratory rate and work of breathing, and improves alveolar ventilation.

Clinical uses

In the acute setting, the two principal indications for NIV are acute exacerbations of COPD and acute cardiogenic pulmonary oedema. However NIV may be considered in other conditions, e.g. chest wall deformity and neuromuscular disease, decompensated sleep apnoea, chest trauma, asthma, pneumonia and to assist weaning in the intensive care unit; expert advice should be sought.

Chronic obstructive pulmonary disease

Consider using NIPPV in patients with an acute exacerbation of COPD, an acute respiratory acidosis (pH < 7.35; H^+ > 45 nmol L^{-1}), and who remain acidaemic despite maximal medical treatment on controlled oxygen therapy for no more than 1 hour. Give oxygen to maintain the oxygen saturation of arterial blood between 88% and 92%; an excessive inspired oxygen concentration may increase CO_2 retention. In approximately 50% of patients who are initially acidaemic on arrival in the emergency department, blood gas values will be returned to baseline in response to this treatment.

Despite some case series documenting beneficial effects of CPAP in the treatment of acute exacerbations of COPD, it is conventional practice to use NIPPV in this situation.

Cardiogenic pulmonary oedema

CPAP is widely used for the treatment of patients presenting with acute cardiogenic pulmonary oedema. It improves patient symptoms, physiology and blood gases by the mechanisms outlined above. Rates of intubation, but not mortality, are also reduced. No difference in outcome has been identified between using CPAP or NIPPV in these patients. However, NIPPV may be considered in patients with acute cardiogenic pulmonary oedema who fail to improve with CPAP, particularly if they are hypercapnic.

Patient suitability

Several factors predict success in patients with acute respiratory failure who require non-invasive ventilatory support. These include less severe physiological derangement and less pre-existing comorbidity; an improvement in pH, P_aCO_2 and respiratory rate after 1 hour of NIV; and a high-quality patient-machine interface. Some patients are unable to tolerate tight-fitting facemasks – nasal masks are available, but these are generally less efficient (the patient must be able to keep their mouth closed) and are not commonly used in the acute setting. NIV helmets are available and may be better tolerated. Some patients have difficulty synchronizing their breathing with the NIV system. Facial anatomy influences the success of NIV: edentulous patients may have particular difficulties with a facemask.

Contra-indications

The most important contra-indication to the use of NIV is the need for immediate tracheal intubation and conventional ventilation. Many of the factors previously considered as contra-indications are relative – with experience, the boundaries for the use of NIV are expanding. For example, after application of NIPPV, the neurologically obtunded patient with an acute exacerbation of COPD may quickly become more conscious as the P_aCO_2 decreases. Many contra-indications are negated if tracheal intubation is considered inappropriate and NIV is to be used as the 'ceiling' of treatment. Important contra-indications to NIV include:

- the need for immediate tracheal intubation and ventilation;
- facial trauma or burns;
- fixed obstruction of the upper airway;
- vomiting;
- patient refusal/intolerance.

Relative contra-indications include:

- recent facial, upper airway or upper gastrointestinal tract surgery;
- inability to protect the airway;

- haemodynamic instability (requiring inotropes/vasopressors, unless managed in a critical care unit);
- severe comorbidity;
- impaired consciousness;
- confusion or agitation;
- bowel obstruction;
- copious respiratory secretions;
- undrained pneumothorax.

NIV may be used in these circumstances, particularly if tracheal intubation is not deemed appropriate.

Complications

If patients are selected correctly, the majority of complications are relatively minor. Potential complications of NIV include:

- Hypotension: an increase in intrathoracic pressure reduces right ventricular end diastolic volume and can cause hypotension, particularly if there is hypovolaemia.
- Barotrauma: over-inflation and gas trapping are possible, although pneumothorax is rare.
- Discomfort: patients frequently find the facemask uncomfortable and claustrophobic.
- Gastric distension: although NIV can cause gastric inflation, prophylactic placement of a nasogastric tube is not required in every patient.
- Pulmonary aspiration: vomiting or regurgitation into a tight-fitting facemask may cause massive aspiration.
- Pressure necrosis: this may be prevented by the use of a hydrocolloid or similar dressing placed over vulnerable areas such as the bridge of the nose. This problem is much less common with modern NIV masks.

Environment

Patients treated with NIV should be managed in an environment with suitable monitoring, including continuous pulse oximetry, access to equipment for blood gas analysis, and immediate availability of resuscitation equipment. Staff should be fully trained and experienced in the use of NIV. Personnel skilled in tracheal intubation should be available with minimal delay.

Equipment

Figure 12.1 shows a simple CPAP valve that is easy to use and can deliver almost 100% oxygen.

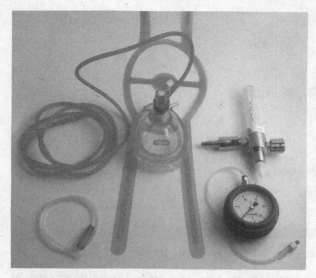

Figure 12.1 A Boussignac valve.

Figure 12.2 shows a typical portable non-invasive ventilator that is able to provide both CPAP and NIPPV. These ventilators were designed initially for home ventilation: they are simple to use and usually portable. However, because air is entrained with high-flow oxygen in an open circuit, it is not possible to measure F_IO_2 or deliver an inspired oxygen concentration of greater than 50–60%.

A more sophisticated ventilator is shown in Figure 12.3. This will provide CPAP and NIPPV with an inspired oxygen concentration of up to 100%. This machine has significant monitoring capabilities, but it is more complicated to use, not portable and significantly more expensive than alternatives.

Interface

Several patient–machine interfaces are available, including nasal masks, facemasks and helmets. The most widely used interface in an emergency setting is the facemask. The mask must be sized and fitted correctly, and not applied too tightly. Most modern NIV machines and masks are designed to allow some leak around the mask to improve patient triggering and tolerance. The correct position of the mask is from just above the chin to the top of the nasal bridge, as illustrated in Figure 12.4.

As an alternative to CPAP, high-flow nasal oxygen therapy is now in common use. High-flow, warmed, humidified air/oxygen mixtures delivered

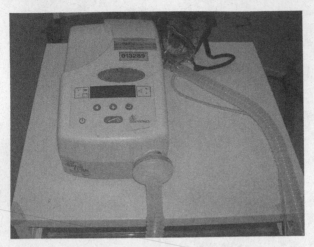

Figure 12.2 Respironics Synchrony non-invasive ventilator.

through nasal cannulae are superior to most standard oxygen delivery systems because they facilitate washout of anatomical deadspace and provide low-level positive airway pressure.

Procedure

General approach to initiating NIV (CPAP or NIPPV)

- Reassure the patient and explain what you are planning to do.
- Select the correct size of facemask.
- With the patient sitting or semi-recumbent, turn on the NIV system and gas flow, set the desired oxygen concentration.
- Apply the mask to the patient's face.
- Patient acceptance may be facilitated if the mask is applied manually for the first few minutes.
- Once the patient is comfortable with the system, apply the straps to produce a snug, but not excessively tight, fit. Ensure there is no significant leak around the facemask.

CPAP (main indication – Type 1 respiratory failure, such as cardiogenic pulmonary oedema):

- Start with a CPAP at 5–10 cmH_2O.
- Titrate F_iO_2 to achieve S_pO_2 of 94–98%.
- If initial CPAP level does not alleviate hypoxia/breathlessness, increase CPAP level to 15 cmH_2O.

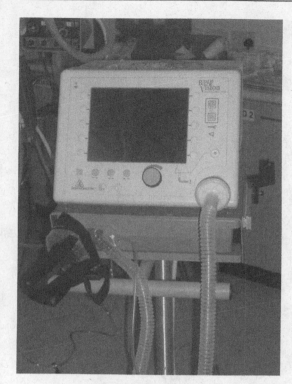

Figure 12.3
Respironics Vision non-invasive ventilator.

- If CO_2 level starts to increase consider NIPPV.

NIPPV (main indication – Type 2 respiratory failure, such as exacerbation of COPD):

- Start with an initial EPAP of 3–5 cmH_2O and IPAP 12–15 cmH_2O.
- Titrate F_iO_2 to achieve S_pO_2 of 88–92% in patients with COPD (or at risk of type II respiratory failure) or 94–98% in other patients.
- Titrate IPAP to patient comfort and CO_2 levels (increase IPAP if remains breathless and/or CO_2 either doesn't improve or worsens).
- Increase EPAP if patient remains hypoxaemic.

Monitoring during treatment

- Observe the patient closely and assess: chest wall movement, coordination of respiratory effort with the ventilator, accessory muscle recruitment,

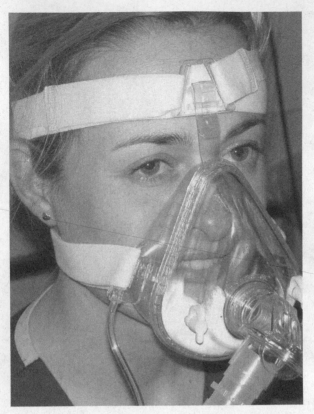

Figure 12.4 Correct mask position for non-invasive ventilatory support.

respiratory rate, heart rate, oxygen saturations, patient comfort and mental state.

- Clinical observations must be recorded every 15 minutes in the first hour and every 30 minutes during the next 4 hours.
- Measure the arterial blood gas values after 1 hour of NIV therapy and after every subsequent change in settings. The frequency of subsequent arterial blood gas analysis will depend on the patient's response to treatment.

Failure of non-invasive ventilatory support

If the NIV optimization manoeuvres described above have not achieved adequate improvement, urgent intubation should be considered. Reassess the patient using the ABCDE approach. Factors suggesting the need for urgent intubation include: airway obstruction, worsening/critical hypoxaemia, laboured respiratory effort, haemodynamic instability and obtunded conscious level.

Consider alternative diagnoses e.g. pulmonary embolism. Next consider whether further specific treatments (e.g. nebulization, vasodilators, chest physiotherapy to aid sputum clearance) are indicated.

If CPAP has produced adequate oxygenation but the patient is tiring and the P_aCO_2 is rising, consider the use of NIPPV or tracheal intubation. A deteriorating P_aCO_2, pH, respiratory rate or conscious level, despite the use of NIPPV, will necessitate an alternative treatment strategy. This might include NIPPV in a timed (mandatory) mode or, if appropriate, tracheal intubation.

Summary

- Consider CPAP for patients with Type 1 respiratory failure, and NIPPV for those with Type 2 respiratory failure.
- Do not use non-invasive ventilation if there is an indication for immediate tracheal intubation, and intubation is appropriate.

Acknowledgements

This chapter has been updated from the first edition chapter, which was written by Alasdair Gray, Jerry Nolan and Carl Gwinnutt.

Figures 12.1, 12.2 and 12.3 supplied by Steve Crane.

Further reading

1   Nava, S., Hill, N. (2009) Non-invasive ventilation in acute respiratory failure. Lancet; 374: 250–9.

2   British Thoracic Society Standards of Care Committee. (2002) BTS guideline: non-invasive ventilation in acute respiratory failure. Thorax; 57: 192–211.

3   Royal College of Physicians/British Thoracic Society. (2008) Non invasive ventilation in chronic obstructive disease: management of acute type 2 respiratory failure. Available at: http://www.rcplondon.ac.uk/resources/concise-guidelines-non-invasive ventilation-chronic-obstructive-pulmonary-disease 2008 report.pdf (accessed December 2013).

4   Agarwal, R., Aggarwal, A.N., Gupta, D., Jindal, S.J. (2005) Non-invasive ventilation in acute cardiogenic pulmonary oedema. Postgrad Med J; 81; 637–43.

5   Gray, A., Goodacre, S., Newby, D.E. et al. (2008) Noninvasive ventilation in acute cardiogenic pulmonary oedema. N Eng J Med; 359(2): 142–51.

Chapter 13

Human factors, audit and skills maintenance

Andrew Burtenshaw, Colin A. Graham and Kevin J. Fong

Objectives

The objectives of this chapter are to:

- Discuss the concept of human factors and their impact on patient safety and clinical effectiveness.
- Describe the development of non-technical skills as a vehicle for positively influencing human factors.
- Provide a framework that identifies personal and organizational weaknesses from a human factors perspective, and supports the development of effective risk reduction strategies.
- Understand the benefit of personal and departmental audit of emergency airway interventions.

Introduction

Every healthcare provider is fallible. Under conditions of time pressure and stress, complex human responses are particularly prone to error. These include impaired perception of elapsed time and decreasing performance in situations associated with excessive cognitive load and rapid task switching.

The challenges of anaesthetizing and intubating critically ill patients, who often have multiple comorbidities, are substantial. Every urgent intubation comprises a series of skilled motor tasks coupled with a significant cognitive load.

The Fourth National Audit Project commissioned by the Royal College of Anaesthetists and The Difficult Airway Society identified a 10-fold increase in the chance of encountering a difficult airway when intubating patients in the emergency department (ED) or the ICU. Urgent intubation and

Emergency Airway Management, Second Edition, ed. Andrew Burtenshaw, Jonathan Benger and Jerry Nolan. Published by Cambridge University Press. © College of Emergency Medicine, London, 2015.

ventilation is required on average 2–3 times per week in urban emergency departments. There are numerous pitfalls to avoid if the patient is to receive optimal care.

Furthermore, medical emergencies are often managed by a team of individuals who have rarely, if ever, worked together before. These challenges emphasize the importance of understanding the non-technical skills that promote good leadership, followership, communication and teamwork in emergency airway management.

Human factors and non-technical skills

Human factors in clinical practice is a discipline which aims to improve clinical performance through an understanding of the impact of teamwork, task prioritization, equipment, workspace, culture, and organization on human behaviour and abilities in the clinical environment. It draws on aspects of human psychology, ergonomics, engineering and environmental sciences.

For acute medicine, the rate at which critical decisions must be made and the complexity of the clinical environment has increased greatly in recent decades. Medicine is not unique in this respect. Other organizations in which technology and risk to human life coincide – most notably the commercial airline industry – have had to face the same challenge and have led the way in investigating human factors and integrating human factors training into everyday practice.

The significant contribution of human factors to a series of aircraft disasters during the 1970s led the National Aeronautics and Space Administration (NASA) to investigate how the non-technical skills of aircrew might be improved. This investigation led to the concept of Crew Resource Management: an approach to teamwork that aims to maximize human resources even when faced with the most difficult scenarios. Initially developed as Cockpit Resource Management, the term was later changed to Crew Resource Management to reflect the contributions of the flight crew, and also those in the wider organization. Translated into healthcare, this concept is commonly referred to as TRM (team resource management). TRM represents a set of specialized non-technical skills that are of relevance throughout everyday processes, not just in the event of an emergency. Indeed, anticipation and limitation of risks is far more effective than reactive crisis management.

Non-technical skills are those skills and behaviours that can be taught or developed and include, amongst others, teamwork (including leadership, followership and communication), situational awareness, decision-making and task management.

It can be helpful to consider human factors at individual, team and organizational levels.

Human factors at the individual level

The individual

All doctors' clinical performances are inconsistent; we all have good days and bad days and are more effective at some times of the day than others. We recognize this ourselves when we are tired or stressed, but more subtle performance deficits go unrecognized. Furthermore, we work in a competitive environment where acknowledging our weaknesses may be counter-cultural. An appreciation of personal limitations enables us to implement mechanisms to address these performance variations, such as asking for assistance, developing effective habits or checking calculations with another practitioner. As individuals we must focus on our weakest performance and develop a working framework where even our least effective performance meets or exceeds the minimum standard.

Physical and mental health

All practitioners will face personal health challenges at some point. Stress contributes significantly to mental overload and can have a considerable impact on an individual's capacity to manage an emergency effectively. It can also influence negatively many non-technical skills, such as the ability to function well within a team, to immediately recall factual information or to maintain situational awareness. Recognizing our own mental overload as well as signs of overload in others is an important skill.

Multi-tasking and the role of habit

When engaged in physical activity that we find challenging, our capacity to think is severely impaired. We are simply not very good at doing two things at once. This affects all elements of cerebral activity, such as strategic thinking, situational awareness and lateral thought, communication or the cognitive processes which help us to integrate within a team. Similarly, intense cognitive workload impairs our ability to carry out physical activity to the best of our ability, although we are usually more aware of this because substandard physical results are more apparent.

Complex clinical practices learnt over a long time may be largely devolved to subconscious, habitual practice: the feeling of performing procedures as 'second nature'. Consigning significant functionality to the subconscious is important as it frees up mental capacity to deal with other aspects of a situation. However, our subconscious mind does not think and adapt; it simply follows learnt patterns according to triggers, which can be diverse and seemingly unrelated. For example, performing a well-rehearsed procedure in an unfamiliar environment can predispose to error simply because the layout of equipment is different, removing an important trigger.

Situational awareness, fixation error, confirmation bias and normalized deviance

Situational awareness (Figure 13.1) is the way in which individuals maintain their perspective while critically important events are happening around them. This can include the passage of time, the changing dynamics of a team, recognizing a changing situation or identifying an alternative course of action. In addition to lateral thought, situational awareness requires anticipation of possible outcomes so that immediate actions can be modified accordingly. This can be described in three stages:

(1) *Detection of cues:* The information taken in and the way in which it is perceived form the basis of interpretation and prediction. This information may present itself in multiple sensory forms from the patient, the team, equipment or the environment. In an airway context, this could include monitor displays and audible alarms, or clinical signs, such as respiratory distress. Incorrect or inadequate cue detection predisposes to incorrect interpretation and prediction.

(2) *Interpretation of the event:* Every individual will assimilate this information slightly differently, according to knowledge, experience and judgement. Confirmation of whether an interpretation is correct may be sought by reviewing whether the cues fit that interpretation. However, it is crucially important that the question being answered is whether there is evidence that the interpretation is *incorrect* in order to avoid confirmation bias (see below). Incorrect interpretation will impair the correct anticipation of possible outcomes.

(3) *Prediction:* Anticipation of possible outcomes allows time for preparation or for preventative measures to be taken. Again knowledge, experience and judgement are called upon, but correct anticipation is reliant upon correct detection and interpretation of cues. Where a situation develops in a way that was not predicted, the available cues and their interpretation must be reconsidered, as this is often an indication of an error at one of these earlier stages.

> Example: During prolonged attempts at a difficult intubation a clinician fails to recognize the duration of hypoxaemia before resuming bag-mask ventilation. They may have exhibited a loss of awareness of time, important physiological parameters or hints from other team members and may have failed to recognize that the goal should have changed from achieving intubation to restoring oxygenation.

A specific example of failed situational awareness is *fixation error* (Figure 13.2), in which a problem has been identified and persistent attempts are made to address it. This interpretation might be incorrect or other priorities might have emerged as the situation unfolds, yet the operator remains fixed on their original interpretation of the situation and its priorities. For example: repeated attempts at intubation when alternative methods of oxygenation

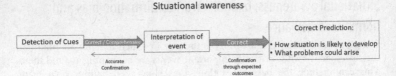

Figure 13.1 Situational awareness.

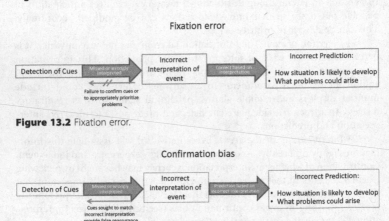

Figure 13.2 Fixation error.

Figure 13.3 Confirmation bias.

are indicated. Fixation error can be transferred to others by communicating either the interpretation (which is incorrect) or the cues (as erroneously detected and interpreted) to a helper as they arrive at a critical situation. To help avoid this, a second practitioner should be aware of the need to re-evaluate the situation from the initial stages.

A loss of situational awareness can also occur when cues are actively sought to match the presumed diagnosis or scenario, while cues that contradict it are ignored. This is known as *confirmation bias* (Figure 13.3), and if based on an incorrect premise, will result in false reassurance. Take care to critically review your own interpretation, particularly when the subsequent course of events fails to match the predicted clinical course, such as if a patient fails to respond to treatment in the way that is expected. Mitigate the risk of confirmation bias by consciously seeking cues which contradict the current conclusion, not just those that favour it. Taking time to review the known facts of the clinical case with other team members can be very helpful in this context.

Normalized deviance (Figure 13.4) describes a situation in which events that should be regarded as abnormal, or outside of accepted standards, become accepted as routine. This can arise through regular exposure to

Normalized deviance

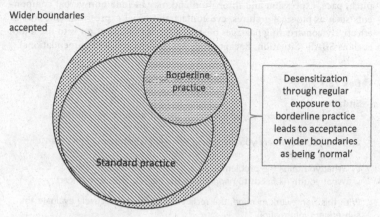

Wider boundaries accepted

Borderline practice

Standard practice

Desensitization through regular exposure to borderline practice leads to acceptance of wider boundaries as being 'normal'

Figure 13.4 Normalized deviance.

borderline or unacceptable standards, and results in a desensitization to the abnormality of the situation. The deviation in practice or standards becomes accepted as normal and is a major contributor to latent risk factors.

Human factors at the team level

Emergency clinical teams (e.g. cardiac arrest team, trauma team, etc.) often comprise a diverse group of individuals interacting for the first time. An effective team makes the best use of its members' skills, communicates calmly and effectively, and is led by an experienced team leader. The leader maintains an overview, picking up on cues from the situation and the team members, and delegates practical interventions to team members, except in rare situations where their experience is required, e.g. creating a surgical airway. A good team leader will empower and encourage all members of the team to contribute to decision-making and will listen to and consider all suggestions. Team leaders are also responsible for influencing the hierarchy. A strict authoritarian leadership approach ensures that instructions are followed, but is usually unresponsive to input from other team members and does not foster good team dynamics. The most effective teams have a less vertical hierarchy and are able to take and receive information whilst simultaneously working towards a common goal, adopting a more vertical hierarchy only when necessary.

Communication

Verbal communication requires clear, unambiguous speech, is influenced by pitch, pace, expression and intonation and may include non-verbal components such as physical gestures, eye contact and facial expression. One way of effectively constructing passages of speech for communication is to use a tool such as SBAR (Situation, Background, Assessment and Recommendations).

Box 13.1

Situation:
  The opening sentence, which frames the subsequent conversation.
  For example:
- Who you are, where you are calling from and which patient you are calling about.
- What you think the problem is.
- What you think needs to happen or what help or advice you need.

With this framework in mind, the recipient can more effectively evaluate the subsequent information.

Background:
  Significant elements of the patient's background. For example:
- Age, gender
- Presenting complaint and medical history
- Functional capacity

Assessment:
  Assessment of the situation. For example:
- Vital signs
- Clinical examination findings

Recommendations:
  What you think needs to happen. For example:
- I think I need your assistance with this potentially difficult airway...
- I'd like your advice on this management plan...
- I think the patient needs... (Procedure/imaging etc.)

Closed loop communication

Under stressful, fast moving and noisy conditions, it is very easy for important elements of communication to be missed, or misinterpreted. Closed loop communication involves repetition of the instruction by the recipient to the issuer. For example, during a cardiac arrest, the practitioner responsible for injecting adrenaline repeats back 'Give 1 mg adrenaline IV' in response to the instruction to do so. A variation of this can also be useful during telephone conversations where a summary at the end of the conversation would include a list of key decisions and actions that have been agreed.

Human factors at the organizational level

Organizational culture

Organizations delivering healthcare play a major part in the development of safe and effective patient care. External organizations (e.g. specialty associations or colleges) enhance safety by disseminating information through communication networks and through their influence on training.

Standardization of tasks and checklists

Standardizing tasks and eliminating clinical practice that falls outside or near the boundaries of accepted practice reduces error rates.

Standardization of tasks determines acceptable practice and creates auditable standards. The ability to acknowledge and follow standardized processes, yet adapt and respond flexibly to unexpected events, is a key element of effective TRM.

Checklists standardize task implementation; effective examples include the World Health Organization's operating room checklist and the Matching Michigan campaign. Emergency intubation checklists are now used commonly.

Critical incident reporting and reflective learning from error

Critical incident reporting is the means by which risks can be identified, monitored and managed. Critical incident reporting must be followed by fair evaluation and sharing of knowledge through effective feedback.

Technology and device design

Medical equipment rarely fails. Errors usually result from the interaction of individuals with the equipment, emphasizing the importance of effective medical device training and uniformity of equipment across clinical areas. Some technology, such as electronic prescribing, may also provide opportunities to mitigate risk.

Latent risk factors

Latent risk factors are the factors present in processes or work environments that permit error. Multiple barriers to error reduce the risk (e.g. equipment checks), but will each carry their own potential for error or latent risk factor. When these opportunities for error coexist within a situation a clinical error takes place. This concept is described as the Swiss cheese model (Figure 13.5).

Latent risk factor identification facilitates effective process change to mitigate that risk.

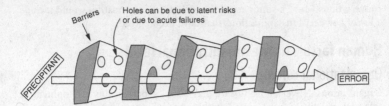

- Failure of multiple barriers allows a precipitant to develop into an error.
- Risk can be reduced by
    - increasing the number of barriers.
    - reducing the number of latent risks and acute failures (number of holes).
    - reducing the potential for error (reducing the size of the holes).
    - ensuring latent risks do not occur under the same conditions (taking the holes out of alignment).

Figure 13.5 The Swiss cheese model (adapted from Reason, J. (2008) *The Human Contribution*. Farnham: Ashgate).

Training and simulation

High-fidelity simulation is particularly effective for human factors training. Some training schemes now include specific educational assessments, such as the Anaesthetic Non-Technical Skills (ANTS) assessments, and increasing use of simulation facilities encourages individuals and teams to become immersed in scenarios enabling human interactions to be reviewed and developed. In contrast to real patient encounters, simulation enables specific scenarios to be explored on demand without the risk of causing patient harm. This provides the freedom to make mistakes and learn from them in a non-threatening, supervized environment.

Audit and skills maintenance

Principles of clinical audit

Clinical audit is the monitoring of specific interventions against agreed standards of care, facilitating the identification and investigation of problems so that solutions can be implemented and their impact reaudited.

Clinical audit can also be used to drive a quality improvement process for a department or hospital. The resources, process and outcome of emergency airway care can all be audited.

Personal audit

Every practitioner should maintain a personal record of emergency airway interventions, which can be presented as an indication of experience achieved.

Departmental audit

Departmental audit facilitates quality control, and ensures that all emergency airway practitioners are achieving an acceptable standard. It also highlights any equipment or staffing deficiencies, e.g. the availability and use of waveform capnography for all intubations.

Skills maintenance

Skills maintenance in emergency airway management can be difficult because of infrequent exposure, particularly with difficult airways. Simulation or regular sessions in operating rooms can help bridge this gap.

Interdepartmental interfaces

Effective interdepartmental collaboration with respect to airway management facilitates:

- safe and effective airway management using multispecialty teams;
- safe and effective interdepartmental transfer;
- an effective airway training, audit and governance programme.

The majority of patients intubated in the ED will subsequently require critical care support making early involvement important. The critical care team is also usually involved in transfers both within and between hospitals.

It is also important to maintain effective interfaces with other departments such as anaesthesia, surgery, radiology, paediatrics and ENT, as these are all commonly involved in the subsequent care of patients requiring emergency airway management.

Summary

- Human factors are major determinants of the outcome of clinical activity.
- Prevention is better than an emergency response.
- Non-technical skills influence behaviour and may be learnt to improve personal risk management. These skills include teamwork, communication, situational awareness, decision-making and task management.
- Organizational factors also have a big impact on risk management.
- Personal and departmental audit together with skills maintenance are important in emergency airway management.

Acknowledgement

This chapter includes updated text from the first edition written by Jerry Nolan, Mike Clancy, Jonathan Benger and Colin Graham.

Further reading

1 Carthey, J., Clarke, J. *The 'How To' Guide: Implementing Human Factors in Healthcare*. Patient Safety First Campaign. Available at: www.patientsafetyfirst.com (accessed November 2013).

2 Reason, J. (1990) *Human Error*. Cambridge: Cambridge University Press.

3 Van Beuzekom, M., Boer, F., Akerboom, S., Hudson, P. (2010) Patient safety: latent risk factors. Br J Anaesth; 105: 52–9.

4 Clinical Human Factors Group website. www.CHFG.org (accessed November 2014).

5 Bion, J.F., Abrusci, T., Hibbert, P. (2010) Human factors in the management of the critically ill patient. Br J Anaesth; 105: 26–33.

Appendix 1 Mnemonics

```
P
E
A
C
H A V N O
    M   H
    P   E
    L   L
    E   P O P E S
```

PEACH: Checks before rapid sequence induction of anaesthesia

Positioning

Equipment – including drugs

Attach – oxygen and monitoring

Checks – resuscitation, brief history, intravenous access and neurology

Help – who is available and what are the abilities of the team?

HAVNO: An aide-memoire for airway assessment

History – including previous airway problems

Anatomy – features of the face, mouth and teeth that may suggest
   intubation will be difficult, and trauma suggesting anatomical
   disruption or blood in the airway

Visual clues – obesity, facial hair, age and trauma (e.g. blood in the airway)

Neck – neck mobility and accessibility, including the presence of in-line
   stabilization

Opening of the mouth – less than three fingers' breadth suggests potential
   difficulty with intubation

AMPLE: Important information to acquire before anaesthetic induction

Allergies

Medications

Past medical history

Last . . . anaesthetic? (complications), meal?, tetanus?

Events leading up to this situation

O HELP!: Useful considerations following a failed initial attempt at intubation

Oxygenation
Head elevation
External laryngeal manipulation
Laryngoscope blade change
Pal – call for assistance

POPES: Common causes of hypoxaemia during invasive ventilation

Position of tube (oesophageal or bronchial intubation; tube out of trachea)
Obstruction (obstructed tubing, tracheal/bronchial obstruction or broncho-constriction e.g. severe asthma)
Pneumothorax (particularly tension pneumothorax) or pleural effusion
Equipment (incorrect kit or connections/equipment failure/inadequate gas flow)
Splinting (abdominal distension including stomach distension or poor paralysis)

Appendix 2 Emergency airway algorithms

Acknowledgement

Martin Wiese designed the visual layout of algorithms 2.1 and 2.3. Algorithm 2.2 is an adaptation based on the layout by Martin Weise.

Guidelines are also available from the Difficult Airway Society at http://www.das.uk.com (accessed November 2014).

Assessing urgency

Planning for intubation

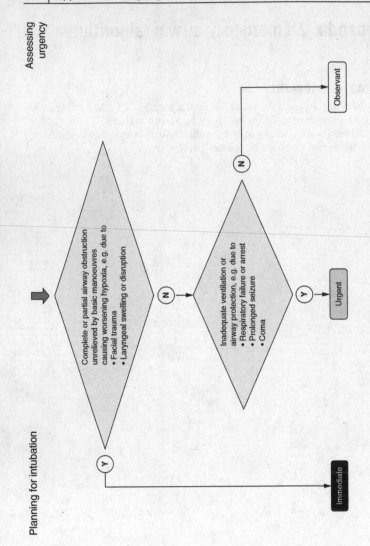

Complete or partial airway obstruction unrelieved by basic manoeuvres causing worsening hypoxia, e.g. due to
• Facial trauma
• Laryngeal swelling or disruption

Y → Immediate

N →

Inadequate ventilation or airway protection, e.g. due to
• Respiratory failure or arrest
• Prolonged seizure
• Coma

Y → Urgent

N → Observant

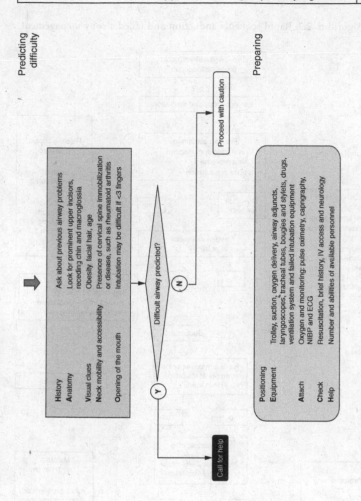

Algorithm 2.1: Patient assessment and preparation for intubation.

Predicting
difficulty

History	Ask about previous airway problems
Anatomy	Look for prominent upper incisors, receding chin and macroglossia
Visual clues	Obesity facial hair, age
Neck mobility and accessibility	Presence of cervical spine immobilization or disease, such as rheumatoid arthritis
Opening of the mouth	Intubation may be difficult if <3 fingers

Difficult airway predicted?

Y — Call for help

N — Proceed with caution

Preparing

Positioning	
Equipment	Trolley, suction, oxygen delivery, airway adjuncts, laryngoscopes, tracheal tubes, bougies and stylets, drugs, ventilation system and failed intubation equipment
Attach	Oxygen and monitoring: pulse oximetry, capngraphy, NIBP and ECG
Check	Resuscitation, brief history, IV access and neurology
Help	Number and abilities of available personnel

Algorithm 2.2: Rapid sequence induction and failed airway management

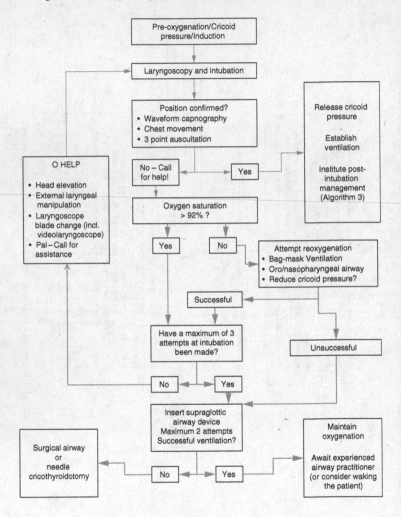

Pre-oxygenation/Cricoid pressure/Induction

↓

Laryngoscopy and intubation

↓

Position confirmed?
- Waveform capnography
- Chest movement
- 3 point auscultation

No – Call for help! ← Yes → Release cricoid pressure

Establish ventilation

Institute post-intubation management (Algorithm 3)

O HELP
- Head elevation
- External laryngeal manipulation
- Laryngoscope blade change (incl. videolaryngoscope)
- Pal – Call for assistance

Oxygen saturation > 92% ?

Yes   No

→ Attempt reoxygenation
- Bag-mask Ventilation
- Oro/nasopharyngeal airway
- Reduce cricoid pressure?

Successful ←

Have a maximum of 3 attempts at intubation been made?

Unsuccessful

No ← Yes

Insert supraglottic airway device
Maximum 2 attempts
Successful ventilation?

No   Yes

Surgical airway or needle cricothyroidotomy ←

Maintain oxygenation

Await experienced airway practitioner (or consider waking the patient)

Algorithm 2.3: Post-intubation management

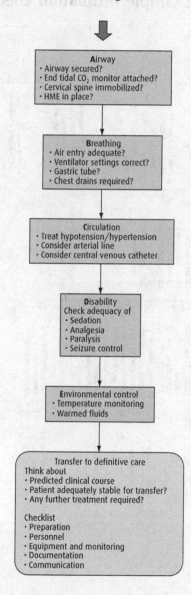

Airway
· Airway secured?
· End tidal CO_2 monitor attached?
· Cervical spine immobilized?
· HME in place?

Breathing
· Air entry adequate?
· Ventilator settings correct?
· Gastric tube?
· Chest drains required?

Circulation
· Treat hypotension/hypertension
· Consider arterial line
· Consider central venous catheter

Disability
Check adequacy of
· Sedation
· Analgesia
· Paralysis
· Seizure control

Environmental control
· Temperature monitoring
· Warmed fluids

Transfer to definitive care
Think about
· Predicted clinical course
· Patient adequately stable for transfer?
· Any further treatment required?

Checklist
· Preparation
· Personnel
· Equipment and monitoring
· Documentation
· Communication

Appendix 3 Example intubation checklist

EMERGENCY INDUCTION CHECKLIST

Prepare Patient

- Is preoxygenation optimal?
  - ETO₂ > 90%
  - Consider CPAP

- Is the patient's position optimal?
  - Consider sitting up

- Can the patient's condition be optimised any further before intubation?

- How will anaesthesia be maintained after induction?

Prepare Equipment

- What monitoring is applied?
  - Capnography
  - SPO₂ probe
  - ECG
  - Blood pressure

- What equipment is checked and available?
  - Self-inflating bag
  - Working suction
  - Two tracheal tubes
  - Two laryngoscopes
  - Bougie
  - Supraglottic airway device

- Do you have all the drugs required?
  - Consider ketamine
  - Relaxant
  - Vasopressor

Prepare Team

- Allocate roles;
  - Team leader
  - First Intubator
  - Second Intubator
  - Cricoid Pressure
  - Intubator's Assistant
  - Drugs
  - MILS (if indicated)
  - Rescue airway

- How do we contact further help if required?

Prepare for difficulty

- If the airway is difficult, could we wake the patient up?

- What is the plan for a difficult intubation?
  - Plan A: RSI
  - Plan B: e.g. BMV
  - Plan C: e.g. ProSeal LMA
  - Plan D: e.g. Front of neck

- Where is the relevant equipment, including alternative airway?
  - DO NOT START UNTIL AVAILABLE

- Are any specific complications anticipated?

This Checklist is not intended to be a comprehensive guide to preparation for induction

RTIC Severn

Reproduced with permission from John Wiley & Sons, Inc.
Reference: Nolan, J. P., Kelly, F. E. (2011) Airway challenges in critical care.
Anaesthesia, 66: 81–92.

Appendix 4 NAP4 Summary: major complications of airway management in the United Kingdom

Fourth National Audit Project of The Royal College of Anaesthetists and The Difficult Airway Society (NAP4): implications for emergency airway management outside the operating room

Tim Cook, Nick Woodall, Chris Frerk and Jonathan Benger

Introduction

The Fourth National Audit Project of the Royal College of Anaesthetists and Difficult Airway Society (NAP4) was a large programme of work designed to identify and study serious airway complications occurring during anaesthesia, in intensive care units (ICU) and in emergency departments (ED) in the United Kingdom. It reported in March 2011, and the full report is freely available online. It is essential reading for all airway practitioners, and there are a number of important learning points relevant to emergency airway management outside the operating room.

Methodology of NAP4

Reports of major complications of airway management (death, brain damage, emergency surgical airway, unanticipated ICU admission and prolonged ICU stay) were collected from all National Health Service hospitals over a period of 1 year. An expert panel reviewed inclusion criteria, outcome and airway management to ensure the correct cases were included and to maximize the amount that could be gained from each, and identified key themes and learning points.

Overall Results

A total of 184 events met inclusion criteria: 36 of these occurred in the ICU and 15 in the ED. In ICU, 61% of events led to death or persistent neurological injury; in the ED 31% of events resulted in these outcomes. Airway events in the ICU and the ED were more likely than those during anaesthesia to occur out-of-hours, be managed by doctors with less anaesthetic experience and lead to permanent harm. Failure to use capnography contributed to 74% of cases of death or persistent neurological injury. The project findings suggested that avoidable deaths due to airway complications occur in both the ICU and the ED. Secondary analysis suggested events may be at least 30 times more common in the ED than during anaesthesia.

Key Themes from the NAP4 Report

The following themes, of particular relevance to emergency airway management outside the operating room, were identified:

- Analysis of the cases identified gaps in care that included: poor identification of at-risk patients; poor or incomplete planning; inadequate provision of skilled staff and equipment to manage events successfully; delayed recognition of events; failed rescue due to lack of, or failure of interpretation of, capnography.
- Failure to use capnography in intubated patients undergoing positive pressure ventilation likely contributed to more than 70% of ICU related deaths and also contributed to deaths in the ED. Mandating the use of capnography in all invasively ventilated patients was identified as the single change with the greatest potential to prevent deaths such as those reported to NAP4.
- As well as ensuring that continuous waveform capnography is present and used, practitioners must be able to interpret the capnograph trace in critical illness and injury. In more than one case reported to NAP4 the lack of a capnograph trace was attributed incorrectly to cardiac arrest, when in fact a somewhat attenuated, but typical, trace can be seen in cardiac arrest whilst cardiopulmonary resuscitation (CPR) is ongoing (Figure 1). The possibility of incorrect tube placement was therefore not considered. This problem was also identified in events occurring during anaesthesia, and raises the possibility that there is a deficiency in current training on this topic. Understanding this issue is directly relevant to any practitioner managing the airway in an emergency.
- Most events in the emergency department were complications of rapid sequence induction. This was also an area of concern in the ICU. Rapid sequence induction outside the operating room requires the same equipment and support that is provided during routine anaesthesia. This includes waveform capnography and immediate access to the equipment needed to manage routine and difficult airway problems.
- Clinicians managing the airway outside the operating room more frequently failed to follow recognized protocols or pathways for managing airway complications. This included repeating techniques and omission of

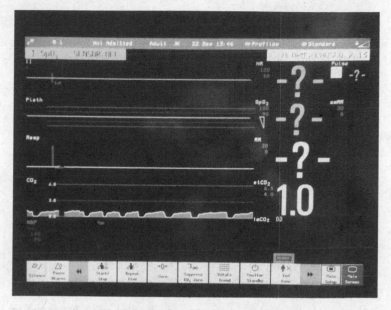

Figure 1 Capnograph trace during cardiac arrest with CPR in progress (reproduced by kind permission of Simon Chapman).

basic procedures. Individuals involved included those, such as anaesthetists, who might be expected to use these pathways in their 'normal environment'. However, even when used correctly, rescue techniques appeared to fail more often outside the operating room. Awareness of these human and technical challenges is important.

- Airway management is a fundamental anaesthetic responsibility and skill; anaesthetic departments should provide leadership in developing strategies to deal with difficult airways throughout the entire organization and this includes regular communication with ICU and ED staff in this regard.

Recommendations from NAP4

- Base emergency department airway management on the concept of the right person, right place, right equipment and right preparation. These concepts are described in detail in the full report.
- The ICU and ED should have available for immediate use a difficult airway trolley broadly the same as that in the operating room. This should be stocked, maintained and checked regularly.

- Good and ongoing communication between senior clinicians in the emergency department, anaesthesia, critical care, ENT and other relevant specialties is essential in planning for, and managing, the emergency airway problems that present to the emergency department. Consider designating consultant leads from each involved specialty to agree and oversee the management of emergency airway problems presenting to the emergency department.
- Ensure agreed plans are in place for the management of all common and predictable emergency department airway emergencies.
- Establish robust processes to ensure the prompt availability of appropriately skilled and senior staff at any time of the day or night to manage the airway within a reasonable timeframe.
- All practitioners who may be called upon to manage airway emergencies outside the operating room must have the required skills and experience, with immediate access to senior supervision. This is particularly important for trainees in emergency medicine and critical care.
- The authors advocate the use of a pre-intubation checklist and an example is provided in Appendix 3.

Conclusions

At least one in four major airway events in a hospital are likely to occur in the ICU or the ED. The outcome of these events is particularly adverse. Analysis of the cases in NAP4 identified repeated gaps in care that include: poor identification of at-risk patients, poor or incomplete planning, inadequate provision of skilled staff and equipment to manage these events successfully, delayed recognition of events, and failed rescue due to a lack of, or failure of interpretation of, capnography. NAP4 indicated that avoidable deaths due to airway complications occur during emergency airway management outside the operating room, and airway practitioners must take proactive steps to avoid these problems in their hospitals and clinical practice.

Further Reading

1   Cook, T., Woodall, N., Frerk, C. (eds.). (2011) Fourth National Audit Project of The Royal College of Anaesthetists and The Difficult Airway Society. Major complications of airway management in the United Kingdom. Report and findings. London: The Royal College of Anaesthetists. ISBN 978–1-9000936-03-3. Available at: http://www.rcoa.ac.uk/system/files/CSQ-NAP4-Full.pdf (accessed July 2014).

2   Cook, T., Woodall, N., Harper, J., Benger, J. on behalf of the Fourth National Audit Project. (2011) Major complications of airway management in the UK: results of the

Fourth National Audit Project of the Royal College of Anaesthetists and the Difficult Airway Society. Part 2: intensive care and emergency departments. Br J Anaesth; 106(5): 632–42. Available at: http://bja.oxfordjournals.org/content/106/5/632.full.pdf+ttp (accessed July 2014)

3   Further resources such as presentations and webcasts are available at the NAP4 home page: http://www.nationalauditprojects.org.uk/NAP4_home#pt (accessed July 2014).

Index

Printed in the United States
By Bookmasters